DIEPSS

A second-generation rating scale for antipsychotic-induced extrapyramidal symptoms: Drug-induced Extrapyramidal Symptoms Scale

Toshiya Inada, M.D.

Seiwa Hospital,
Institute of Neuropsychiatry

Seiwa Shoten Publishers
Japan 2009

DIEPSS
A second-generation rating scale for
antipsychotic-induced extrapyramidal symptoms:
Drug-induced Extrapyramidal Symptoms Scale

Author: Toshiya Inada, M.D., Ph.D.
　　　　Associate Professor
　　　　Department of Psychiatry and Psychobiology
　　　　Nagoya University, Graduate School of Medicine
　　　　65 Tsurumai-cho, Showa-ku, Nagoya-shi,
　　　　Aichi 466-8550, Japan
　　　　E mail: toshiya.inada@gmail.com

Published by Seiwa Shoten Publishers, Inc.,
1-2-5 Takaido, Suginami-ku, Tokyo 168-0074
Tel +81-3-3329-0031(Sales Department)
　　 +81-3-3329-0033(Editorial Department)
Fax +81-3-5374-7186

First published on September 17, 2009
Second printing on October 3, 2016
Printed in Japan
Typesetting by Image Brains Inc., Tokyo

ISBN 978-4-7911-0722-3

© Toshiya Inada,M.D.
All rights reserved. No part of this publication may be reproduced,
stored in a retrieval system, or transmitted, in any form or by any
means, electronic, mechanical, photocopying, recording, or otherwise,
without the prior permission of the publisher or the author.
Permission is granted for reproduction for use by researchers and clinicians.

CD-ROM entitled "DIEPSS Evaluation Training Sheet (5 languages versions) ver 1.1" has been typeset by Image Brains Inc., Tokyo, and published by the Japanese Society of Psychiatric Rating Scales (JSPRS) in Tokyo, Japan, on October 20, 2008.
For order of the CD-ROM, inquiry as to the training workshop using the video-recorded material authorized by the Japanese Society of Psychiatric Rating Scales (JSPRS), contact to: info@jsprs.org
Image Brains Inc., The editorial office of the Japanese Society of Psychiatric Rating Scales (JSPRS), 3-23-8 Hacchobori, Chuo-ku Tokyo 104-0032, Japan

Contents

Foreword I
Preface 1
1. Process of Development of the DIEPSS 2
    1.1. Before the development of the DIEPSS in Japan 2
    1.2. Suspension of the development of a Japanese version of the SAS 3
    1.3. Suspension of the development of a Japanese version of the ESRS 4
    1.4. Establishment of the DIEPSS 5
    1.5. Advantage of using the DIEPSS 7
2. General comments for using the DIEPSS 9
    2.1. Each evaluation should be made independently 9
    2.2. The highest anchor point should be chosen 9
    2.3. The severest symptoms should be evaluated 10
    2.4. Repeat evaluations should be made at the same time of day. 10
    2.5. How to handle the rating '1 (minimal, questionable)' 10
    2.6. How to handle EPS not of drug-induced origin 11
    2.7. Differentiation between the continuous and intermittent states. .. 11
3. DIEPSS Individual Items 12
    3.1. Subclassification 12
    3.2. Parkinsonism 13
        3.2.1. Gait 14
        3.2.2. Bradykinesia 15
        3.2.3. Sialorrhea 17
        3.2.4. Muscle rigidity 18
        3.2.5. Tremor 19
        3.2.6. Differential Diagnosis 20
    3.3. Akathisia 21
        3.3.1. Clinical features 22
        3.3.2. Differential diagnosis 22
    3.4. Dystonia 23
        3.4.1. Clinical features 24
        3.4.2. Differential diagnosis 25
    3.5. Dyskinesia 25
        3.5.1. Clinical features 25
        3.5.2. Differential diagnosis 26
    3.6. Overall Severity of Extrapyramidal Symptoms 27
4. Reliability of the DIEPSS 28
    4.1. Inter-rater Reliability 28
        4.1.1. Japanese study 28
        4.1.2. Korean study 30
    4.2. Test-retest Reliability 30
        4.2.1. Japanese study 30
        4.2.2. Korean study 31
    4.3. Training Utilities 31
5. Validity of the DIEPSS 32
    5.1. Factor Structure 32
        5.1.1. Japanese study 32
        5.1.2. Korean study 33

    5.2. Concurrent Validity 33
        5.2.1. Correlation between the DIEPSS and other EPS scales 33
        5.2.2. Comparison with western scales in a double-blind study of olanzapine 34
    5.3. Evaluation of Optimal Cut-Off Scores 34
    5.4. Predictive Validity 35
6. Clinical application of the DIEPSS 37
    6.1. Comparison of EPS profiles between typical and atypical antipsychotics 37
        6.1.1. Comparison of EPS profiles between olanzapine and haloperidol 37
        6.1.2. Comparison of EPS profiles between olanzapine and fluphenazine 38
        6.1.3. Comparison of EPS profiles between quetiapine and haloperidol 38
        6.1.4. Comparison of EPS profiles between aripiprazole and haloperidol 40
        6.1.5. Comparison of EPS profiles between blonanserin and haloperidol 41
    6.2. Preventive Strategies for EPS using the DIEPSS 43
    6.3. Other clinical and biological studies 43
        6.3.1. Quetiapine treatment for behavioral and psychological symptoms of dementia (BPSD)
        in patients with senile dementia of the Alzheimer type (SDAT) 44
        6.3.2. Correlation between reduction of EPS and improvement in quality of life (QOL) ... 44
        6.3.3. Association between antipsychotic-induced EPS and polymorphisms in the dopamine
        D2-receptor (DRD2) gene 44
        6.3.4. Serum testosterone levels and the severity of negative symptoms 45
References 46

Appendix i
    I. Japanese version ii
    II. Chinese version vi
    III. Taiwanese version x
    IV. Korean version xiv
    V. English version xviii

Foreword

I would like to take this opportunity to congratulate Dr. Inada on the publication of this English manual for his DIEPSS. It has been repeatedly pointed out that the first-generation scales for evaluation of extrapyramidal signs and symptoms available in English are not optimal from various viewpoints. Dr. Inada, a world renowned expert in clinical psychopharmacology based in Japan, tackled this problem head-on and developed the DIEPSS in 1994. The Japanese manual was published in 1996.

Not only did Dr. Inada develop the DIEPSS, but also made invaluable videoclips available to aid the teaching of the ratings of extrapyramidal signs on the basis of the DIEPSS. He has carried out more than 100 workshops on the evaluation of extrapyramidal symptoms, and the responses from the participants have helped Dr. Inada to fine-tune the teachings of the DIEPSS itself. The net result is the DIEPSS itself, which has excellent psychometric results and unprecedentedly rich learning aids. I recommend its wider use around the globe.

May 17, 2009

Toshi A. Furukawa, M.D., Ph.D.
Professor and Chair, Department of Psychiatry and Cognitive-Behavioral Medicine, Nagoya City University Graduate School of Medical Sciences, Nagoya, Japan

◆◆◆

I have followed the development of the Drug-induced Extrapyramidal Symptoms Scale (DIEPSS) by Dr. Inada for almost 15 years. The DIEPSS is based on careful selection of individual items. The scale has been thoroughly tested and the data show that it has high validity and reliability. Dr. Inada has extensive experience with the training of clinicians (I have witnessed his training course in Hungary), which is reflected in the excellently described, precise instructions and in the simplicity of the scale.

The DIEPSS is the most extensively studied rating scale for measurement of antipsychotic/neuroleptic-induced extrapyramidal symptoms. This book gives a detailed description of the DIEPSS, which I highly recommend for all those working in the field of extrapyramidal symptoms and rating scale development. The book will be helpful to those teaching others about extrapyramidal side effects, and also for researchers who have to assess these symptoms in the course of their studies. I hope that the scale will become widely used internationally and will help to improve the safety of antipsychotic drug use.

May 22, 2009

Istvan Bitter, M.D., Ph.D., D.Sc.
Professor and Chair, Department of Psychiatry and Psychotherapy, Semmelweis University, Budapest, Hungary

◆◆◆

It is my great pleasure that the English manual of the DIEPSS is now being published. I wish this could have happened earlier, considering the design of the instrument and the implications of accurate assessment of EPS profiles in patients receiving antipsychotic agents.

The DIEPSS has an excellent training system that includes videoclips showing various severities

Foreword

of DIEPSS. In my opinion, the DIEPSS training seminar is actually not only important for obtaining high inter-rater reliability, but it can also be seen as a chance for young psychiatrists to understand the fundamental symptomatology of drug-induced EPS. As detailed EPS scales were developed during the era of typical antipsychotics (which were associated with a higher incidence of EPS), the DIEPSS may be one of the standard EPS rating instruments, specifically designed for the side effects profile of second-generation antipsychotics.

I sincerely hope that the EPS characteristics in patients receiving the next generation of antipsychotics will be extensively studied using this scale, and that it may contribute to better understanding of the EPS features of the next generation of antipsychotics.

May 24, 2009

Norio Ozaki, M.D., Ph.D.
Professor and Chair, Department of Psychiatry, Nagoya University Graduate School of Medicine, Nagoya, Japan

◆◆◆

The English manual for the Drug-induced Extrapyramidal Symptoms Scale (DIEPSS), developed by Dr. Inada, has finally been published. Although the initial design of this scale was created in Japan, Dr. Inada completed it during his period of clinical research at McLean Hospital, Harvard Medical School. In that sense, the "hometown" of this scale is the United States of America. It must have been developed for international use. The DIEPSS was established in 1994 and its Japanese manual was published in 1996. It has been used for 15 years in Japan and is an indispensable scale for studies of drug development and clinical research on antipsychotics in Japan.

The evaluation of extrapyramidal symptoms in Europe and America has been done mainly with a combination of the Simpson and Angus Neurological Rating Scale for evaluation of parkinsonism, the Barnes Akathisia Scale for evaluation of akathisia, and the Abnormal Involuntary Movement Scale for evaluation of dyskinesia. Thus it has been inconvenient for raters to use three different scales at the same time. On the other hand, the DIEPSS is a very simple scale to use because it consists of only nine items for overall evaluation of extrapyramidal symptoms.

In contrast to other medical fields that consider physical diseases, no objective biological markers have been identified in the psychiatric field, and clinical symptoms are the only signs that can be used for the diagnosis and evaluation of psychiatric diseases. Therefore, rating scales play an essential role in the evaluation of symptoms in clinical psychiatry research. Scales are required to have not only high reliability and validity, but also a simple design, a relatively short time for evaluation, clear and intelligible anchor points, and well-organized training materials. The DIEPSS fulfills all of these requirements.

Psychiatric rating scales used in Japan have mostly been developed outside Japan, and then translated into Japanese. Although we have thus depended on such scales developed overseas, I believe that the DIEPSS is an excellent rating scale we can be proud of, and can recommend it for use outside Japan.

May 25, 2009

Teruhiko Higuchi, M.D., Ph.D.
President, National Center of Neurology and Psychiatry, Kodaira, Japan

◆◆◆

Foreword

As an old friend and colleague of Dr. Toshiya Inada, I have had the pleasure of working with him on various collaborative research projects at the Division of Psychopharmacology, Department of Neuropsychiatry, Keio University School of Medicine. Skilled at generating innovative ideas, Dr. Inada has made remarkable achievements in a broad range of research related to psychiatric disorders, including molecular genetics and clinical pharmacology. Today, he is a leader in the field of psychopharmacology in Japan.

Dr. Inada has long been interested in the side effects of antipsychotic drugs, devoting his efforts in particular to the prevention of tardive dyskinesia. He created the Drug-induced Extrapyramidal Symptoms Scale (DIEPSS), an unparalleled scale that enables precise assessment of the severity of drug-induced extrapyramidal side effects of antipsychotic drugs. The DIEPSS has become the standard scale used in clinical trials on new antipsychotic drugs in Japan.

The DIEPSS is used worldwide as a practical, standard rating scale matched to assessment of extrapyramidal symptoms. In recent years, it has also been used in international collaborative clinical trials led by Japan, and is being used in various Asian countries.

The publication of this book, which explains the DIEPSS in depth, thus comes at a very opportune time. It is my sincere hope that this book will further increase the awareness of the DIEPSS in the psychopharmacological community, promoting its use in an even greater number of countries and helping it to develop into a truly international scale.

May 28, 2009

Shigenobu Kanba, M.D., Ph.D.
Chairman and Professor, Department of Neuropsychiatry, Graduate School of Medical Sciences, Kyushu University, Fukuoka, Japan

❖❖❖

It would be an excellent idea for Dr Inada to introduce the English manual for the DIEPSS to the world. Dr Inada graduated from Keio University and has been studying the side effects of antipsychotic agents, especially extrapyramidal symptoms (EPS), throughout his career. He conducted a large-scale prospective study of tardive dyskinesia for which earned his doctoral degree. He established the new rating scale for EPS through repeated evaluation of a large number of schizophrenic patients.

The DIEPSS was established in 1994, when Dr. Inada was studying at McLean Hospital, Harvard Medical School, Boston, and was awarded a Rafaelsen fellowship for his prominent research activities in this field at the 19th annual meeting of the Collegium Internationale Neuro-Psychopharmacologicum held in Washington DC, USA. In recent years, his research interests have expanded to the molecular genetics of psychiatry, including genetic vulnerability to tardive dyskinesia. In 2008, he won another award, the academic encouragement award of the JSCNP Dr. Paul Janssen Research Award from the Japanese Society of Clinical Neuropsychopharmacology for his outstanding research in this field.

Dr. Inada has compiled the fruits of many years of study of the DIEPSS into this book. I think this represents the beginning of a new era of the disputable evaluation strategy of EPS profiles. I anticipate that this scale will be used throughout the world, and will become a valuable tool for clarifying the remaining unsolved clinical issues in this field.

May 31, 2009

Haruo Kashima, M.D., Ph.D.

Foreword

Professor and Chairman, Department of Neuropsychiatry, Keio University School of Medicine, Tokyo, Japan.

❖❖❖

In clinical trials of antipsychotics, evaluations of their extrapyramidal side effects, as well as their main effects on the positive and negative symptoms of schizophrenia, are crucial. Several scales for evaluating the severity of extrapyramidal movements have been developed and used for clinical trials, but clinicians are eager to use simpler, more sensitive and more reliable scales. Dr Inada has developed a new scale, the DIEPSS, which meets these expectations. This scale has already been used in many clinical trials and has been widely acclaimed by both pharmaceutical companies and clinicians in Japan.

Now, Dr. Inada has published an English language version of the DIEPSS instruction manual. Publication of this version has been long awaited ever since the DIEPSS was developed, but I believe that the time taken for it to appear reflects the great care that has gone into its compilation. I anticipate that this scale will be used worldwide and will be of great public benefit.

June 2, 2009

Masaomi Iyo, M.D., Ph.D.
Professor and Chairman, Department of Neuropsychiatry, Chiba University Graduate School of Medicine, Chiba, Japan.

❖❖❖

It is good - to say nothing of reassuring - to see researchers continuing the work of refining the way we assess and record drug-related movement disorders and I applaud your detailed efforts, clearly the result of many years of experience and endeavour. Alas, many psychiatrists allowed themselves to become 'blinkered' to the problem and accepted without criticism the largely industry-sponsored view that EPS were a thing of the past. Would that this were true! They are still there for those with a keen eye to see and remain a key issue in clinical management. The implication is that monitoring should once again become a mantra for clinicians prescribing antipsychotic drugs and the best way to monitor is to gain expertise in standardised rating.

The whole area of rating scales in this field has however become fossilized, with a few early pioneers continuing to dominate. This might have happened because the early scales were prefect but, like you, I believe that this was not the case. The tools we have had available to us in the past have fundamentally fallen short on the task demanded of them by failing to capture adequately the diversity and pervasiveness of the issues. Thus, your contribution to the field is to be welcomed as a soundly clinically-based and statistically refined alternative that attempts to address the weaknesses of previous scales.

June 19, 2009

David Cunningham Owens, M.D., Ph.D.
Professor of Clinical Psychiatry, University of Edinburgh, Scotland, United Kingdom

Preface

This book is designed as an official detailed commentary on the Drug-induced Extrapyramidal Symptoms Scale (DIEPSS) for precise assessment of the severity of drug-induced extrapyramidal symptoms during treatment with antipsychotic drugs. The DIEPSS is widely used as a practical, standard rating scale matched to the extrapyramidal symptom (EPS) profiles of current second-generation antipsychotics, which are characterized by clinical simplicity, excellent sensitivity, and high reliability.

The DIEPSS is recommended not only as a screening instrument in the outpatient mental clinic to facilitate detection of early manifestations of EPSs, but also as a tool for differentiating the EPS profiles of any new antipsychotic agent from those of conventional ones in double-blind randomized controlled trials.

This book is divided into six parts: The first part introduces the historical and psychiatric background to the development of the DIEPSS. The second and third sections give a detailed commentary on the DIEPSS and a guide to its usage. Each EPS is delineated on the basis of individual items in the DIEPSS so that clinicians can easily become accustomed to the use of this scale. The fourth and fifth sections describe the results of previous validity and reliability studies, which have demonstrated the excellent sensitivity and high reliability of this scale. The final section describes the clinical application of the DIEPSS to psychopharmacological studies in which EPSs were evaluated using this scale.

Although the prevalence of EPSs has decreased since the introduction of second-generation antipsychotics, some patients still have a high risk of EPSs and often develop severe EPSs during treatment with these drugs. The EPSs develop as a result of central nigrostriatal dopaminergic antagonism, and there is no antipsychotic compound that lacks antidopaminergic activity. Therefore, clinical psychiatrists should always be aware of the potential risk of EPSs during antipsychotic treatment. I expect that this book will be of interest to clinicians who are seeking the best available method for evaluation of these side effects.

The author is sincerely grateful to Dr Gohei Yagi, Dr George Gardos, Dr David Cunningham Owens and Dr Istvan Bitter for their valuable comments, and to Dr. Yong Sik Kim, Dr. Shih-Ku Lin and Dr. Qiuqing Ang for translation into their native languages.

May 10, 2009

Toshiya INADA, M.D., Ph.D.

1. Process of Development of the DIEPSS

1.1. Before the development of the DIEPSS in Japan

The advent of antipsychotic drugs such as chlorpromazine and haloperidol brought about an epoch-making advance in the treatment of schizophrenia. However, it also gave rise to a new clinical problem: extrapyramidal symptoms (EPS) were very frequently observed during the administration of these first-generation agents, and this greatly influenced the development of further antipsychotic drugs.

In the era of first-generation antipsychotics, it became clear that it was important to evaluate in minute detail the severity of a variety of phenotypes of EPS. During this period, a number of rating scales for evaluating the severity of these conditions were developed, and these have been used in western countries ever since. For example, the Simpson-Angus Scale (SAS), developed by Simpson & Angus (1970), is a neurological rating instrument which focuses exclusively on rating the severity of parkinsonism. This scale was widely used in clinical trials in the treatment of schizophrenia, usually in combination with the Barnes Akathisia Scale (BAS) (Barnes, 1989), a 4-item scale for akathisia, and the Abnormal Involuntary Movement Scale (AIMS) (Guy, 1976). The AIMS was introduced by the National Institute of Mental Health in response to the need for a simple and widely acceptable method for recording drug-induced hyperkinetic movements, and has been used as an independent rating scale for tardive dyskinesia (Guy, 1976). The Japanese version of the AIMS was established in 1977 and was used in the prospective study on tardive dyskinesia (Inada et al, 1991). Subsequently, our research group examined the reliability of, and established, a Japanese version of the BAS (Inada et al., 1996). Chouinard et al (1980) also developed the Extrapyramidal Symptoms Rating Scale (ESRS) to evaluate the global symptomatology of EPS.

In clinical studies evaluating the efficacy of antipsychotic drugs conducted in Japan up until the early 1990s, standardized scales such as the Brief Psychiatric Rating Scale (BPRS) were used for rating the symptomatology of psychosis, but interest in adverse reactions seemed to be relatively low. In practice, no particular standardized scale was used for rating EPS, and serious EPS were picked up as adverse events by the investigators, based on their own judgment. However, this method of rating introduces the risk of divergence among investigators in recognizing and recording cases. It is therefore necessary to rate drug-induced EPS using a standardized scale in order to accumulate objective and reliable data.

With these factors and social demand as the background, the DIEPSS was developed in 1994 for the purpose of rating EPS observed in psychiatric patients receiving antipsychotic medication (Inada & Yagi, 1995, 1996). The development of the DIEPSS began by verifying existing drug-induced extrapyramidal symptoms rating scales, and attempting to establish Japanese versions of these scales. In the first half of the 1990s, various drug-induced extrapyramidal symptoms rating scales were being used in different regions of the world, particularly in western countries, in clinical trials for the treatment of schizophrenia. These were mostly either a combination of the SAS+BAS+AIMS, or the ESRS. However, due to the difficulties outlined in the following sections, the idea of establishing Japanese versions of the SAS and ESRS was abandoned in favor of producing a new rating scale.

Thanks to the introduction of newer atypical antipsychotic agents, which have more favorable EPS profiles than conventional antipsychotic agents, drug-induced EPS are unlikely to be as great a source of concern as previously. However, some patients are still at high risk for EPS and therefore clinicians should take an interest in the emergence of EPS in patients receiving antipsychotic agents. With these factors in mind, a practical, standardized rating scale, which is brief, simple and easy to administer, has been sought in recent clinical psychopharmacological research. The DIEPSS was designed to fulfill this role in a manner which makes it suitable for international use.

1.2. Suspension of the development of a Japanese version of the SAS

There are two types of rating scale for evaluating EPS: one is the combined scale, developed to evaluate global EPS manifestations including parkinsonism, akathisia, dystonia and dyskinesia. Such scales include the ESRS and the St. Hans EPS. The other type of scale is designed to focus exclusively on a particular symptom such as parkinsonism (SAS), akathisia (BAS) or dyskinesia (AIMS). Unless one specific symptom is the focus of interest, the combined use of rating scales for individual symptoms, for example the SAS+BAS+AIMS, or one of the scales for rating global EPS, for example the ESRS, can be used to grasp the overall EPS profile.

Of these, the SAS is the most commonly used rating scale for evaluating drug-induced parkinsonism in clinical psychopharmacological research in western countries, and it was also used as a standard comparison scale in a previous study on the validity of the EPS rating scale (Loonen et al., 2000). It consists of 10 individual items, and has been considered to be the most representative scale of the typical antipsychotic era. The initial metric profiles of the reliability and validity of this scale were reported in 1970 (Simpson & Angus, 1970). A number of modified versions have since been developed. In an attempt to establish a Japanese version, each of the individual items of the SAS was reviewed. As a result, our research group was confronted with the following difficulties:

(1) It is often pointed out that the scale structure is weighted heavily on items rating rigidity. Of the total of 10 items, 6 are devoted to the evaluation of rigidity, while there is only one item for evaluating bradykinesia. Thus, with a view to evaluating parkinsonian symptoms comprehensively and uniformly, the validity of this scale may be lacking and should be re-established in the translated version.

(2) Various items relating to muscle rigidity and glabellar tap are unlikely to be characteristic drug-induced EPS that psychiatrists would consider clinically important in the early stages of antipsychotic treatment. From this standpoint, the scale does not appear to capture the most clinically appropriate parkinsonian side effects well.

(3) Since the severity of the items relating to muscle rigidity cannot be visualized, for example by video imaging, a true assessment of severity is only possible when one sees an actual patient for oneself. However, sets of patients exhibiting each of the levels of severity described by the anchor points could not be recruited for the reliability study. Therefore, for practical purposes, it is impossible to confirm inter-rater reliability for all of the anchor points before starting a clinical trial. When it comes to test-retest reliability, at least half of all the items cannot be assessed.

(4) Another factor that must be addressed from the viewpoint of clinical psychiatry is the kind of EPS that influence the acceptability of antipsychotics to the patients receiving them. Since the SAS focuses exclusively on parkinsonian symptoms, it is natural that items concerning akathisia, dystonia and dyskinesia are not included. However, acute dystonic reactions, such as tongue protrusion and oculogyric crisis, and/or the strong, subjective inner restlessness of akathisia seen during the early stages of antipsychotic treatment often lead to reluctance to take antipsychotic medication, potentially resulting in non-adherence and, ultimately, relapse of the psychosis.

Besides the adverse impact of early-onset EPS on drug compliance, the motor symptoms caused by dystonia and the dyskinesia that is seen after prolonged use of antipsychotic agents are often undetectable in the early stages of antipsychotic treatment, but delays in detecting these conditions may have long-term consequences. They can often persist as treatment-resistant movement disorders even after the discontinuation of antipsychotic medications.

On the other hand, while the muscle rigidity and/or bradykinesia caused by antipsychotics are generally considered to be side effects, in the clinical setting, they may complement the sedative effects of antipsychotics in patients who are markedly restless or agitated. In other words, from the standpoint of clinically significant symptoms that cause patients the most distress – and from the standpoint of being able to develop a meaningful rating scale for side effects that allows one to quantify the level of distress in the clinical setting – it is essential that not only items relating to parkinsonism, but also those relating to akathisia, dystonia and dyskinesia, should be included as items that absolutely must be assessed in schizophrenic patients receiving antipsychotics.

Ultimately, since there were several critical issues with the validity of the SAS as an index for assessing the severity of side effects in the field of psychiatry, and it would be difficult to establish its reliability in the actual clinical setting, the research plan for validating the Japanese version had to be abandoned.

The author organized a symposium entitled "Neuroleptic associated tardive syndrome: clinical features and neuropathology" at the 19th Collegium Internationale Neuropsycho- Pharmacologicum held in Washington, D.C., in 1994. At this symposium, it was pointed out that there is no rating scale for drug-induced extrapyramidal symptoms that could be considered fully appropriate and of satisfactory usefulness, and the necessity of developing such a scale was stressed.

Subsequently, Dr. Owens of the University of Edinburgh stated the following opinion regarding the SAS in the book "A guide to the extrapyramidal side-effects of antipsychotic drugs," published in 1999 by Cambridge University Press.

> "The Simpson-Angus Scale is not possessed of the psychometric properties that might redeem this widely used scale from its manifest inadequacies. For 4 of its items, the mean inter-rater correlations in the original publication are below 0.66, with ranges from as low as 0.16, and only glabellar tap, the least valuable and probably valid sign in drug-related disorder, has a mean coefficient above 0.80. The persistence of this scale must not be interpreted as an endorsement of the excellence with which it performs the task required of it. It is, in fact, a reflection of sterility in the field of scale development over the past quarter century. The Simpson-Angus Scale was a noble pioneer, but now deserves a decent burial. Few clinicians, and no researchers, should shed any tears at its passing. The Simpson-Angus Scale has also become psychiatry's 'Lego' scale, to be built on and demolished by individual workers on the basis of their individual studies of the moment. Indeed, no scale in the history of medicine has been so ruthlessly beaten up and mutilated, yet still refused to die. Such 'modifications' are too numerous to mention but, despite their frequent appearance in the literature, the principle cannot be condoned. Unless such manipulations result in a new instrument of proven clinical and statistical merit, the value of the data provided by the hybrid is of dubious scientific merit, based as it is on little more than a shared name. Merely adding the prefix 'modified' does not alter this fact."

1.3. Suspension of the development of a Japanese version of the ESRS

Subsequent to the review of the SAS, we also reviewed the possibility of establishing a Japanese version of the ESRS, originally developed by Chouinard & Ross Chouinard (1980). This scale is a comprehensive EPS assessment tool which was used in the clinical studies of the atypical antipsychotic risperidone in the treatment of schizophrenia. Since this scale was developed in the era of typical antipsychotic drugs, it contained a total of 31 rating items, including 12 questionnaires for patients.

In the first half of the 1990s, the 18-item Brief Psychiatric Rating Scale (BPRS) was still in wide use for assessing psychiatric symptoms as an index of efficacy. Some experts were of the opinion that, in clinical trials, careful consideration should be given to whether the number of items evaluating adverse events should be more than the number evaluating efficacy. Consequently, it was concluded that it would probably not be possible to introduce a new scale for rating side effects that had more items than the scale used for rating psychiatric symptoms. Moreover, since investigation of each of the rating items in the ESRS involved severity assessments based on up to 9 rankings, with adjectives for expressing severity, it was thought that, without additional specific anchor points, it would be difficult to obtain satisfactorily reliable data in actual use, even if reliability testing were conducted. For these reasons, the validation of the Japanese version was suspended.

Subsequently, it was pointed out that the reliability and validity of this scale had not been investigated sufficiently, even though the manual for the ESRS has recently been published (Chouinard & Margolese, 2005). In addition, the ESRS is a rather lengthy and complex scale for regular use. The length of a rating scale is an important issue which could affect its utility in the clinical and research settings (Martinez-Martin et al, 1994). It may be more desirable to construct a scale that is composed of fewer, but equally reliable, items (Martinez-Martin et al, 1994; Rabey et al, 1997). Dr. Owens of the University of Edinburgh stated the following opinion regarding the clinical issues surrounding the ESRS rating items in the book we cited earlier: "A guide to the extrapyramidal side-effects of antipsychotic drugs," published in 1999 by Cambridge University Press.

"The ESRS is a unique instrument in including 12 questionnaire items to identify subjective symptomatology, a most important innovation in the field. Eight items are devoted to parkinsonian signs, under which is included akathisia (the subjective element is noted in the questionnaire), each rated on a seven-point continuum. This scale once again does not resolve the dilemma of whether it is 'core' symptomatology that should be the target of rating or regional manifestations of 'core' disorder. Thus, bradykinesia is rated conceptually, but so, too, are facial mask and arm swing on separate items.

An attempt to provide for specific ratings of both acute and chronic dystonia is laudable, but frankly does not work. The severity of acute dystonia appears to be judged on the basis purely of signs, which, as has been seen, is inadequate, and although in the original draft one could record dystonia (acute or chronic) of the lips, there was no provision for recording truncal disorder, though this has now been rectified. The major confusion, however, lies in the fact that a number of the descriptions of disorder to be rated under 'dyskinesias', which supposedly refers to non-dystonic hyperkinesias, are clearly dystonic.

The scale does bring a novel approach to the question of comparative judgment in rating hyperkinetic disorders. The question relates to the relative rating one gives mild but persistent disorder versus that for signs that are intermittent but moderate or marked in severity. The ESRS's solution is to recommend rating on the dual axes of frequency and amplitude. This has clear merit for tremor, but whether this extends to choreiform-type hyperkinesias is unclear. Furthermore, how disorder of internal musculature, such as of the larynx, can be graded by these principles is a mystery to the present author. The reasonable implication that this 'dual axis' method of rating will enhance reliability has not been established to date.

The ESRS is also a complex scale for regular use and not all its worthy efforts in the direction of innovation are satisfactory. Its statistical properties appear good but, somewhat surprisingly, these have not been established to quite the level one would expect of such a major instrument (Chouinard et al., 1980; 1984)."

1.4. Establishment of the DIEPSS

After the establishment of the Japanese versions of SAS and ESRS was suspended, the development of a new scale was initiated by our research group in 1992. Firstly, the authors began to collect and review possible individual rating items. These were selected by referring to medical textbooks or academic references on psychopharmacology, in addition to various previously established rating scales for EPS. In developing the new EPS scale, the following points were taken into consideration: It should be useful in the clinical psychopharmacological research. It should be era-matched, that is, as simple as possible and containing the minimum number of absolutely necessary rating items, since the widespread use of second-generation antipsychotic agents was anticipated, and these have a lower incidence of EPS than first-generation antipsychotics. In addition, it should be a sensitive and reliable scale which would be robust enough for advanced scientific and clinical research. The development of the new EPS scale focused especially on the following points:

(1) It was developed as a simple rating scale suitable for capturing the extrapyramidal symptoms associated with second-generation antipsychotic agents, but which would make it possible to assess all of the representative extrapyramidal symptoms seen in the field of psychiatry, that is, to assess parkinsonism, akathisia, dystonia and dyskinesia as drug-induced extrapyramidal symptoms.

(2) For the severity of each item, in addition to the ability to express severity as a summarizing adjective (0: None; 1: Very mild; 2: Mild; 3: Moderate; 4: Severe), all possible efforts were made to include more descriptive explanations of anchor points applying to specific conditions.

(3) For the items relating to motor symptoms such as tremor and dyskinesia, videoclips of specific patients exhibiting severe symptoms were prepared, in order to allow the rater to confirm the level of severity and differences in the nature of the movements by reference to a standardized case.

(4) The rating item for "bradykinesia" in the Keio University extrapyramidal symptom rating scale consisted of the 3 items "gait," "facial expression" and "speech disturbance", but an attempt was made to incorporate "facial expression" and "speech disturbance", which had low inter-rater consistency, into a "bradykinesia" item that included hypokinesia symptoms, and to describe well-defined anchor points. Since the hypokinesia symptoms in the "bradykinesia" item were sometimes hard to distinguish from negative symptoms or symptoms of depression, they were stratified using anchor points that included "facial expression" and/or "speech disturbance" levels of severity. It was decided that, of those items that fell under the heading "bradykinesia," the characteristic parkinsonian gait, which is not affected by negative symptoms or symptoms of depression, would be assessed using the item "gait," independent of "bradykinesia," and it was therefore established as a rating item independent of bradykinesia, with its own specific anchor points.

(5) "Salivation etc" was included among the "other" items in the Keio University extrapyramidal symptom rating scale. However, these "other" items were apt to be rated vaguely. For this reason, the "other" item was deleted from the new scale. Since "salivation" exhibits a high level of provisional consistency with other parkinsonian items, such as tremor and muscle rigidity, it was included as an independent item describing parkinsonism.

Through a process of conducting exhaustive examinations and trying drastic changes such as replacing rating items with a low consistence rate among raters, and by introducing anchor points to improve the consistence rate, etc., a completely new scale was established. Using this draft of the DIEPSS as a base, the rating items and the method of rating were subjected to further extensive study. The final version of the DIEPSS was established in 1994, when the author was working as a visiting researcher at McLean Hospital, Department of Psychiatry, Harvard Medical School, Massachusetts, USA, under the supervision of Dr. George Gardos. Here, the original English version of the DIEPSS was developed. The Japanese version of the DIEPSS was developed simultaneously. Since the original English terms in the DIEPSS were specifically selected so that comparable Japanese terms did exist, the exact Japanese translation was included under each original English sentence for the convenience of Japanese raters.

In establishing a Japanese translation of any rating scale developed in a western country, it is necessary to carry out back-translations. However, even after repeated forward- and back-translation, very often a Japanese version of a scale cannot be made absolutely faithful to the original because there are some English expressions that are difficult to translate into Japanese, or even cannot be translated into Japanese. Likewise, there are some Japanese expressions that cannot be converted into English. However, unlike other rating scales such as the Positive and Negative Syndrome Scale (PANSS) (Kay et al., 1991) and the Brief Psychiatric Rating Scale (BPRS) (Overall & Gorham, 1962), these translation issues could be avoided from the outset for the DIEPSS.

Since the original English text of the DIEPSS was compiled by the Japanese author by selecting English words that correspond exactly with Japanese words, not only in the rating scale itself but also in the DIEPSS user's manual, a faithful Japanese translation is provided in addition to the original text for Japanese raters.

In December 1995, a research proposal entitled "Evaluation of drug-induced EPS", an international collaborative research project with Semmelweis University in Hungary (Hungarian chief investigator: Dr Istvan Bitter), was adopted as an "Inter-Government Collaborative Research on Science and Technology between Japan and Hungary," and in 1996, a budget measure was taken by the Science and Technology Agency in Japan and clinical research using the original version of the DIEPSS (English version) was conducted.

In addition to the Japanese and English versions, a Korean version was established in 2002. Metric profiles of the reliability and validity of the Korean version have been reported (Kim et al, 2002). In 2004, in a comparative study between olanzapine and fluphenazine in post-traumatic stress disorder (PTSD) patients with conducted in Croatia, the DIEPSS was used to assess EPS (Pivac et al, 2004). Subsequently the DIEPSS was also translated into 2 Chinese versions (Simplified Chinese for People's Republic of China and Traditional Chinese for Taiwan) in 2008.

1.5. Advantage of using the DIEPSS

A systematic and reliable assessment of drug-induced EPS is essential in psychiatric research and practice (Barnes & Kane, 1994). Furthermore, a quantitative rating of EPS is indispensable for clinical studies in which the safety and tolerability of antipsychotic drugs are to be evaluated (Conley, 2001). In addition, an accurate assessment of EPS using a standardized rating scale with proven reliability and validity can assist clinicians in evaluating the emergence, severity and subtype of EPS, and in following the changes that occur during treatment (Barnes & Kane, 1994). One of the advantages in using the DIEPSS is that high inter-rater reliability can be easily obtained using the established DIEPSS training system. The DIEPSS video-recorded training material was established in 2001, and a total of 114 training seminars were conducted during the period from September 2001 through August, 2009; these comprised 110 seminars in Japan and 1 in each of the USA, the People's Republic of China, Korea and Taiwan. Using this educational material, video footage supplementing the descriptions of specific anchor points make it possible to learn from visual images that go beyond words. The results of data analyses from raters who participated in these seminars using the DIEPSS video images demonstrated that a high degree of international inter-rater reliability can be easily obtained. In fact, this scale has been confirmed to be a clinically useful rating scale for which a high level of inter-rater reliability in rating EPS in psychiatric patients receiving antipsychotic drugs is ensured.

Another advantage of using the DIEPSS in the evaluation of EPS is its conciseness, simplicity and sensitivity. Although the DIEPSS is composed of only 9 items, including 8 individual items and one global rating, it has been demonstrated that, using this scale, the EPS profiles of first- and second-generation antipsychotic drugs can be clearly distinguished. Following the wide-spread introduction and use of second-generation antipsychotic drugs, which are known to have a significantly lower incidence of EPS than first-generation antipsychotics, the number of patients who develop severe EPS has become significantly smaller. However, concern about drug-induced EPS still remains, and should not be ignored in daily clinical practice. Therefore, accurate ratings of EPS are very important, as well as accurate and comprehensive methods of monitoring changes in psychiatric symptoms.

In 2008, the Japanese Society of Psychiatric Rating Scales (JSPRS) (URL: http://jsprs.org) issued a 5-language CD-ROM of the DIEPSS (English, Japanese, Chinese, Korean and Taiwanese). In recent years, the DIEPSS has also been used in several international collaborative clinical trials of second-generation antipsychotic drugs conducted in the East Asian countries, including Korea, the People's Republic of China, Taiwan and Japan. The DIEPSS is widely used as a simple, concise, sensitive, reliable and valid multidimensional rating scale for drug-induced EPS in schizophrenic subjects treated with antipsychotic drugs, and can be utilized as a combined rating scale in clinical research and practice.

Given the now relatively low incidence of EPS in schizophrenic patients receiving second-generation antipsychotic drugs, EPS scales with many items, such as the ESRS or combined use of the SAS, BAS and AIMS, may be considered too burdensome for general use. Unlike the SAS or the ESRS, which are so-called first-generation EPS scales designed to record the high level of EPS seen with first-generation antipsychotics, the DIEPSS is a second-generation EPS scale; its simplicity and high reliability make it suitable for assessing the low incidence of EPS in the era of second-generation antipsychotics.

In conclusion, the DIEPSS is a simple, sensitive and reliable rating scale that is appropriately matched to the EPS profiles of current antipsychotic drugs and has become a standard rating scale for the evaluation of EPS in Japan, especially in clinical studies of atypical antipsychotic drugs. The DIEPSS is also recommended as a screening instrument in the outpatient clinic to allow the detection of early manifestations of EPS, because the items included encompass the whole range of EPS, from acute signs seen in the early stages of treatment to tardive dyskinesia.

This scale has now become widely used as a global standard evaluation tool for monitoring EPS in the pharmacological treatment of schizophrenia. In view of its simplicity and practical usefulness, it is expected to gradually replace first-generation EPS evaluation methods such as the ESRS, or combined use of the SAS, BAS and AIMS.

2. General comments for using the DIEPSS

Taking into account the arrival of the era of second-generation antipsychotic drugs, the DIEPSS was designed in as simple and concise a format as possible: 8 essential items (the minimum number considered feasible) were selected as individual items which would allow the precise severity of the antipsychotic-induced extrapyramidal symptoms (EPS) observed in psychiatric patients to be evaluated in as short a time as possible. In addition to these 8 individual items, one global item was also included so that an impression of the overall EPS profile could be obtained.

From the point of view of usefulness in clinical psychiatry, the ideal EPS assessment method should use a scale that evaluates the total range of potential EPS, such as bradykinesia, rigidity, tremor, akathisia, dystonia and dyskinesia (Owens, 1999; Gerlach et al, 1993). The DIEPSS is a multidimensional combined rating scale for quantifying the severity of drug-induced parkinsonism, akathisia, dystonia and dyskinesia, as described in the next chapter. General comments regarding the use of the DIEPSS are introduced here. The purpose of this manual is to maximize the reliability of assessments made with the DIEPSS by standardizing the rating method.

> \<General comments\>
> This scale is designed to evaluate the severity of drug-induced extrapyramidal symptoms occurring during antipsychotic drug treatment, and consists of 8 individual items and 1 global item. Raters should have medical training and have sufficient knowledge of the evaluation of neurological symptoms. They also need to have sufficient training on how to use this scale so that they can reproduce stable data. Raters should evaluate the subject's symptoms principally from direct interview with the subject and from observations during the interview. Raters should also take information obtained from the ward personnel and from relatives into consideration. In evaluating individual items of tremor, akathisia, dystonia, etc., the subject may sometimes report that the symptoms appear only at certain times other than during the evaluation interview, such as after receiving night medication or before sleep. In such cases, the raters should carefully evaluate the severity of symptoms considering the interview with the subject as well as the information obtained from the ward personnel and relatives. The severest symptoms observed within the rating period determined in the individual research protocols (e.g. recent 24 hours, recent 3 days, etc.) should be considered for evaluation. The following glossary represents guidelines for rating the specific items.

2.1. Each evaluation should be made independently

When using the DIEPSS, the key principle of the rating system is to use one rating sheet for each rating, in order to perform an independent evaluation every time. In particular, in a clinical study where a change in severity is investigated in the same patient over time, it is generally a required condition that each investigation should be performed in a blind manner without referring to previous ratings.

2.2. The highest anchor point should be chosen

When two different scores are possible, the highest condition (i.e. the one representing the more severe state) should be chosen. Thus, when the rater is unable to differentiate between two severity ratings, the higher of the two ratings should be recorded as the severity of the item.

2.3. The severest symptoms should be evaluated

This scale is based on a combination of direct interviews, observations during the interview, neurological examinations and information from the patient, his/her family and hospital ward staff. Using all this information, the severest symptoms that occur within the stipulated rating period should be recorded as the scores for the individual items. The severest symptoms cannot always be seen during a rating interview; indeed, an intermittent symptom may be absent at this time. Thus, information obtained from the direct interview, neurological examination, observations by the family and/or the complaints of the patient should also be considered when evaluating the individual items, especially for tremor, akathisia and dystonia. When observations during the interview and the information obtained from the patient and his/her family do not agree, the more severe condition should be recorded as the severity of the item. Information regarding a severe condition can often be easily obtained, for example when the patient complains strongly about akathisia, or there is a severe dystonia and/or dyskinesia that onlookers feel is unsightly.

When rating with the DIEPSS is performed at 1-2 week intervals in a clinical study, the rating period is usually set, and is generally somewhere between the last 3 days and the last week. Using this type of protocol, it is possible to indentify intermittent symptoms; for example, although neither the subjective inner restlessness of akathisia nor its objective motor phenomena may be apparent at the time of rating, the patient may complain that he/she suffers from mild symptoms every night before sleep. It is also possible that transient tremor and/or acute dystonic reactions, such as oculogyric crisis or tongue protrusion, occur only at night, and will therefore not be observed at the time of the rating interview. In such cases, since the rater cannot directly observe the exact symptomatology, he/she should carefully judge whether these complaints are reliable enough to be diagnosed as EPS by conducting a detailed medical interview about the situation when it does occur, and by referring to the information given by the hospital ward staff or family as much as possible.

2.4. Repeat evaluations should be made at the same time of day.

The EPS seen in the acute phase of treatment tend to occur at a time when the blood level of the antipsychotic drug is high. The severity of tardive dyskinesia has also been reported to have a diurnal fluctuation (Hyde et al, 1995). With regard to complaints of akathisia or of motor disorders such as dyskinesia and dystonia, information can easily be obtained from the caregiver or family if the symptoms are severe, but there are some instances where such information cannot be collected. In order to avoid the influence of diurnal fluctuation or the antipsychotic blood level, it is preferable to conduct the DIEPSS rating interview at a fixed time on each occasion, e.g., around 10 o'clock in the morning or 3 o'clock in the afternoon. Diurnal variations should be considered for outpatients whose visiting time for DIEPSS evaluation differs depending on the day. The rater should always record the time of day at which the DIEPSS evaluation is performed.

2.5. How to handle the rating '1 (minimal, questionable)'

The severity of '1 (minimal, questionable)' in the anchor point should be used in the following cases: (1) the symptom is uncertain or doubtful, that is, even if the symptom is present, its severity is minimal, thereby making it very difficult to decide whether it is a true EPS, or (2) when the symptom is regarded as mild, but is observed only intermittently and/or occurs to an almost negligible extent. Since a significant diagnostic definition requires a score of 2 or more for each individual item, symptoms with a severity of '1 (minimal, questionable)' would not be included in a prevalence study. However, this severity is clinically important in detecting the early signs of EPS, which require careful follow-up. Early detection of these minimal symptoms may help prevent their progression by allowing early therapeutic interventions to be introduced.

2.6. How to handle EPS not of drug-induced origin

Raters sometimes misunderstand the rating system for EPS that are present at a baseline assessment, i.e. before the administration of an antipsychotic agent. Because they believe that only drug-induced EPS should be recorded for each item, they rate any non-drug-induced EPS present at baseline as '0 (None, Normal)', "because these EPS can be considered as idiopathic or psychogenic, not drug-induced". This idea is a mistake. Although DIEPSS is a literal abbreviation of Drug-induced Extrapyramidal Symptoms Scale, this scale is not intended for rating drug-induced EPS exclusively, but for rating changes in the severity of EPS during the course of antipsychotic therapy. Differential diagnosis is important. However, it should be noted that, when EPS which are not considered to be drug-induced are observed at baseline, these symptoms should not be rated as '0 (None, Normal)' because their etiological origins cannot be definitely differentiated from their clinical manifestations. They should be scored with regard to the exact severity of their clinical manifestations, in faithful accordance with the rater's manual. Using this value as a baseline, the rater should then observe and rate longitudinally to see how the severity of the EPS changes with the subsequent administration of an antipsychotic drug.

In a clinical study of antipsychotic medications for the treatment of schizophrenia, it is sometimes difficult to decide whether a symptom observed at a particular cross-sectional point is drug-induced or of some other origin, such as idiopathic, senile or psychogenic (involuntary movement). In such cases, the rating of severity should be based on the idea of evaluating 'adverse events' and the rater should not record the score as '0 (None, Normal)', despite the possibility of a non-drug-induced origin. The rater should again rate the severity of the actual symptoms observed, in faithful accordance with the rater's manual.

2.7. Differentiation between the continuous and intermittent states

Raters should differentiate between the continuous state and the intermittent state when evaluating the specific individual items tremor and dyskinesia. When rating tremor, they should base this differentiation on evaluations of severity made as frequently as every 10 seconds, considering the repetitive nature of the motor property. In contrast, when rating dyskinesia, raters should observe it for a longer duration, for example several 10-second periods or several minutes, because of the irregular nature of the motor property.

3. DIEPSS Individual Items

EPS remain a major clinical problem in psychiatry. Most patients, estimated at as many as 75-95%, develop EPS to some extent during the course of antipsychotic therapy (Keepers, 1983). EPS can sometimes be extremely uncomfortable and distressing, and impair normal daily activities, adding an additional burden to the existing psychiatric illness. The appearance of these symptoms can sometimes counteract therapeutic efforts. Firstly, they are a frequent cause of drug noncompliance, leading to relapse, rehospitalization and deterioration of psychosis. In addition, if acute EPS are not properly diagnosed and treated soon after their onset, they can lead to treatment-refractory and often irreversible tardive conditions. Routine monitoring for EPS is one of the most important preventive strategies in terms of the safety of antipsychotic drug treatment, since it enables the physician to detect early, mild symptoms, to introduce proper treatment at an early stage, and ultimately prevent widespread clinical problems.

In this chapter, the clinical features, differential diagnoses and remarks on the evaluation of the most common EPS (American Psychiatric Association, 1997; McEvoy et al, 1996), including tardive dyskinesia (TD), are described according to the 8 individual items and 1 global item of the DIEPSS. The global item (Item 9) is rated by considering the severity and frequency of all the individual items, the extent of subjective distress and the degree of influence on the activities of daily living. Anchor points have been established for each of the 8 individual items and the global item. Evaluations of severity for these 9 items are principally based on objective observations, subjective distress and the degree of influence on activities of daily living, which are highly important factors in evaluating EPS (Owens, 1999; Kim et al. 2002b).

3.1. Subclassification

As shown in **Figure 1**, which illustrates the types of EPS induced by antipsychotic drugs, EPS can have several different manifestations. They can broadly be divided into acute and chronic categories (American Psychiatric Association, 1997). Acute types include parkinsonism, akathisia and dystonia. With longer periods of antipsychotic treatment, late-onset forms of EPS, the majority of which are classed as TD, can be observed. These two categories differ with regard to the time from the initiation of antipsychotic treatment to the onset of symptoms, and in their reversibility, dose-dependency and response to various pharmacological treatments. Acute EPS can begin during the first few days of antipsychotic drug administration. Chronic EPS, which include TD and related tardive syndromes, occur after months or years of antipsychotic drug administration. Different mechanisms are thought to underlie the development of the two categories. The blockade of dopamine D2 receptors in the central nervous system may be involved in the development of acute EPS, while chronic EPS may arise due to the hypersensitivity of dopamine D2 receptors in the central nervous system.

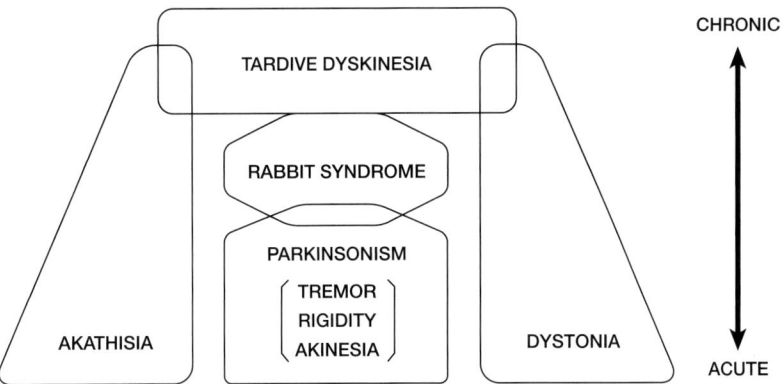

Figure 1. Extrapyramidal symptoms induced by antipsychotic drugs

3.2. Parkinsonism

Parkinsonism occurs in 10-50% of patients treated with therapeutic doses of antipsychotic drugs, and can be observed from the initial phase of treatment (Tarsy, 1983). The symptoms are basically identical to those seen with idiopathic parkinsonism, with the triad of tremor, rigidity and bradykinesia.

The hypokinetic neuroleptic-induced extrapyramidal symptoms of bradykinesia or akinesia may appear as a kind of subtle behavioral disturbance, in which the patient is deprived of initiative, spontaneity or a sense of vitality (Rifkin et al, 1975; van Putten & May, 1978; Siris, 1987). This can easily be misdiagnosed or misinterpreted as a manifestation of depression, negative symptoms or schizophrenic 'burn out'. In very severe cases, it may mimic catatonia. Depressive symptoms have been reported to be present in over 50% of patients with akinesia. The depressive states which appear secondary to akinesia are termed 'akinetic depression', in contrast to the primary psychiatric symptoms of depression. Bradykinesia or akinesia usually responds to a reduction in the antipsychotic dose or treatment with an anticholinergic drug, while antidepressants may be effective for depressive illness.

Section 3. DIEPSS Individual Items

3.2.1. Gait

> <Item 1. Gait>
> Ask the subject to walk as he/she normally would on the street. Rate slowness of gait in this item, namely, the degree of reduction in speed and step, as well as decrease in pendular arm movement. Also consider the degree of stooped posture and propulsion phenomenon. When the intensity of these symptoms does not fit an anchor point, rate giving priority to the severest symptom observed in the subject. The degree of difficulty in initiating and/or terminating walking should also be considered in rating the item of bradykinesia.
>
> 0. Normal.
>
> 1. Impression of minimal reduction in speed and step of gait, and minimal decrease in pendular arm movements.
>
> 2. Mild reduction in speed and step of gait with mild decrease in pendular arm movements. Mild stooped posture is also observed in some cases.
>
> 3. Clearly slowed gait with greatly diminished pendular arm movements. Typical stooped posture and gait with small steps. Propulsion phenomenon is sometimes observed.
>
> 4. Initiation of walking alone is barely possible. Even if gait is initiated, the subject shows shuffling gait with very small steps and no pendular arm movements are observed. Severe propulsion phenomenon may be observed.

A change in gait is primarily classified as a symptom of bradykinesia. For example, the characteristic loss of arm-swing on walking results from the progression of bradykinesia. However, in contrast to the difficulty in differentiating the other hypokinetic EPS associated with bradykinesia (described in the next section) from the retardation of movement associated with depression and affective flattening, the parkinsonian gait is very characteristic and can be easily recognized. Therefore, gait has been adopted as an independent individual item in the DIEPSS, separate from the bradykinesia item. Besides being a typical parkinsonian feature, gait is sensitive for all the clinical signs of antipsychotic-related bradykinesia. Reduction in pendular arm-swing is a frequent and sensitive indicator of antipsychotic treatment. A characteristic gait can be detected in the majority of patients receiving antipsychotic medication, especially in the initial phase of treatment, when their doses are being increased.

Gait disturbance should be evaluated in an open space. In mild cases, walking speed becomes slower and step-length is mildly reduced. Pendular arm-swing also diminishes. When rating the gait, the patient's age should also be considered. If the walking speed is a little slow, but can be regarded as normal considering the age, then it should be rated as 'normal gait'. With the onset of parkinsonism, the arms, instead of moving freely on walking, describe an increasingly restricted arc and are eventually held immobile by the sides. As the condition progresses, a combination of loss of arm-swing with changes in posture is observed. Increasing arm flexion and abduction, usually associated with advancing pronation, also become evident. Subsequently, the arms become permanently flexed and abducted with the knuckles rotated through 90 degrees, thus ending up 'facing the front'. With further increases in the severity of symptoms, gait disturbance becomes apparent in a slowing of pace and a reduction in both the length and the height of the step. The normal sequence of walking usually involves the heel hitting the ground first, followed by the ball of the foot. In mild cases of parkinsonism, the patient initially walks flat-footed. Subsequently, as severity increases, the sequence of walking is inverted to ball-to-heel, with the effect of reducing the forward propulsive force of each step. This combination of an inverted sequence with small, shallow steps gives rise to the characteristic appearance and sound of the shuffling parkinsonian gait. A propulsion phenomenon due to forward momentum also makes patients look as if they are running; this is known as 'festination'. In severe cases, the patient cannot instantly control forward and backward movement, and so may not be able to start or stop voluntarily. This gives rise to anteropulsion when the motion is in a forward direction and retropulsion when it is backwards.

3.2.2. Bradykinesia

> <Item 2. Bradykinesia>
> Reduced activity due to slowness and poverty of movements. Initiating movements is delayed and is sometimes difficult. Rate the degree of poverty of facial expression (mask-like face) and speech during interview (monotonous, slurred speech), as well.
>
> 0. Normal.
>
> 1. Impression of slowness in movements.
>
> 2. Mild bradykinesia. Slowed movements and loss of muscle tone.
>   Slight delay in initiation and/or termination of movements. Mild reduction in facial expression and rate of speech.
>
> 3. Moderate bradykinesia. Clear impairment in initiating and/or terminating movements.
>   Rate of speech is moderately slowed, and facial expression is moderately impaired.
>
> 4. Severe bradykinesia, or akinesia. The subject rarely moves, or moves with great effort.
>   Almost no changes in facial expression (typical mask-like face).
>   Markedly slowed speech.

Bradykinesia means a slowing down of movements ('kinesis' is ancient Greek in origin for movement). It produces a physical state of diminished spontaneity, characterized by a slow gait with small steps, few gestures, and difficulty with initiating usual activities. Lack of facial expression, apathy and a reduction in spontaneous speech can also be observed in patients with this condition. It is one of the most common symptoms of antipsychotic-induced parkinsonism, seen in up to 80% of patients receiving antipsychotic treatment. Bradykinesia (known as akinesia when it is severe) involves a loss or absence of voluntary motor activity. This has 4 principal manifestations: 1) diminution or poverty of background motor activity, 2) slowed execution of movements associated with difficulty in initiation, 3) progressive fatiguing and diminishing amplitude of repetitive alternating movements, 4) an interruption to the flow of consecutive movements (Owens, 1999).

Bradykinesia affecting the facial muscles induces a mask-like face, a condition known as hypomimia (sometimes referred to as amimia), with a characteristic 'flat' facial expression. A reduction in facial expression/speech or frank facial masking results in the subject showing little or no emotion. Patients with bradykinesia may appear somewhat listless or lifeless and their face may lose its usual range of expressions. In this condition, smiling, blinking and spontaneous eye movements are less frequent. In its more severe form, the patient has difficulty frowning, speech is slurred and the lips may be permanently parted. The subtle changes in facial expression normally seen when the patient is thinking, speaking or otherwise communicating disappear, to be replaced with a fixed and relatively immobile face. Graduations in affective display diminish, and the patient often appears somewhat vacant.

In other areas of the body, bradykinesia produces a slowing of or reduction in voluntary movements due to its effect on the systemic musculature. It becomes difficult for the patient to initiate movement; for example, several attempts are sometimes necessary to get out of a chair. Voluntary and spontaneous movements are decreased both in frequency and amplitude. In conversation, there is a lack of interactive posture and gesture, with the individual seeming distant and uninvolved. The ability to perform tasks that demand rapid or complex movements is gradually impaired, and the slowing of movement may ultimately become 'freezing.' Disruption to the flow of consecutive movements may become evident, with actions appearing hesitant and disjointed, or the patient may become incapable of initiating or completing a task.

The slowness and incompleteness of movement can also affect speaking and swallowing. Impaired coordination of the muscles in the mouth and throat may sometimes result in difficulty in swallowing, while poor control of the speech muscles may induce dysarthria. Hypokinetic dysarthria can be characterized by monotony of pitch and volume, reduced emphasis, a variable rate, imprecise consonants, and a breathy and harsh voice. In mild cases, these symptoms can be detected from the patient's complaints, such as "It became difficult to swallow foods", or "I cannot speak clearly". When symptoms of difficulty in swallowing and/or dysarthria are observed in patients receiving antipsychotic medications, the severity of these symptoms should be evaluated in this item, taking into consideration the patient's level of distress and the influence of the impairment on activities of daily living.

<Question 1> How do I rate bradykinesia with a slowed gait?

When rating the bradykinesia item, do I also have to consider the degree of slowing of gait?

Answer 1: As noted in section '3.2.1. Gait', the degree of slowing of gait should be evaluated in the gait item. When the walking speed becomes slower and shaking of the upper limbs reduces, one feels, as a natural course, that movement is giving way to inactivity. In chronic schizophrenic patients with marked negative, depressive or autistic symptoms, it is often difficult to differentiate these from the slowness of movement induced by extrapyramidal bradykinesia, especially in a cross-sectional clinical rating. When rating the bradykinesia item, the rater should consider the degree of difficulty in initiating movements and the degree of poverty of facial expression (mask-like face), which are considered to be peculiar to EPS, and the manner of speech during the rating interview (monotonous, slurred speech). In contrast, when rating the gait item, degrees of reduction in speed and step, and any decrease in pendular arm movement, are evaluated independently of the bradykinesia item, taking into account any characteristic features of EPS such as stooped posture and propulsion phenomena.

3.2.3. Sialorrhea

<Item 3. Sialorrhea>
Rate the severity of excess salivation.

0. Normal.

1. Impression of minimal excess salivation during interview.

2. Mild excess saliva pooling in mouth observed during interview.
   Little difficulty in speaking.

3. Moderate excess salivation observed during interview.
   Often results in difficulty in speaking.

4. Constantly observed severe excess salivation or drooling.

Sialorrhea means excessive production of saliva. In mild cases, the patient may simply have a sensation of moistness in the mouth, but as the symptom progresses, an imbalance between the production and clearance of saliva results in pooling on the floor of the mouth and eventual drooling. Sialorrhea is not considered to be an entirely objective sign. However, it can be a distressing feature of parkinsonism if it becomes prominent, although patients vary considerably in the distress they experience from apparently comparable degrees of abnormality and this affective overlay can make the feature hard to evaluate. In severe cases, the patient may always need to carry a handkerchief in his/her hand.

The pathophysiological basis of sialorrhea is complex. Although the term sialorrhea implies excessive production of saliva, it is unclear whether this offers a universal explanation. Sialorrhea is frequently observed in patients receiving clozapine, a drug with a strikingly reduced liability to induce EPS overall (Owens, 1996). The excess salivation observed in patients receiving antipsychotic agents may also be a result of impaired swallowing secondary to bradykinesia of the oropharyngeal musculature rather than of autonomic origin.

When rating the sialorrhea item, the rater should ask the patient to keep his/her mouth open for certain period of time. When the mouth is kept open, saliva usually accumulates to some extent, even in healthy subjects, as experienced in the dental clinic. The rating of severity should be judged by checking whether the amount accumulated is within or above the normal range.

3.2.4. Muscle rigidity

<Item 4. Muscle rigidity>
Rate the severity of resistance to flexion and extension of the arms. Rate cogwheeling, waxy flexibility, and the degree of flexibility of wrists, as well.

0. Absent.

1. Impression of minimal resistance to flexion and extension of the arms.

2. Mild resistance to flexion and extension of the arms. Mild cogwheeling is sometimes noted.

3. Moderate resistance to flexion and extension of the arms. Obvious cogwheeling may occur.

4. Extreme resistance to flexion and extension of the arms.
   The subject may maintain posture, when interrupted (waxy flexibility).
   Flexion and extension of the arms is sometimes impossible due to extreme muscle rigidity.

Muscle rigidity means stiffness or inflexibility of the muscles. It is defined as an increase in the resting muscle tone that is evident on passive movement, and is observed as a resistance to flexion and extension of the muscles, resulting in difficulties with motor performance. Muscles normally stretch when they move and relax when they are at rest. In rigidity, the muscles of an affected limb are always stiff and do not relax, sometimes resulting in a decreased range of motion. An individual with rigidity may not be able to swing his/her arms when walking because the muscles are too tight. There are 2 types of rigidity associated with extrapyramidal disorders. The first type, 'lead-pipe' rigidity, affects agonist and antagonist muscles equally and results in an even resistance to passive movement throughout the range, like trying to bend a lead pipe. In the second type, appropriately referred to as 'cog-wheel' rigidity, the resistance to movement 'gives' at regular intervals, to be rapidly re-established as the motion is pursued. This conveys a jerky, ragged feel throughout the range of movement. Passive movement of a patient's arm during a physical examination may reveal either the constant resistance of lead-pipe rigidity, or the ratchet-like jerks known as 'cog-wheeling', which can often be elicited by slowly rotating the wrist or bending the elbow through the full range of motion. Although it is widely recognized that cog-wheeling is of prime significance in antipsychotic-induced cases, both types of rigidity are significant and diagnostically important. The earliest signs of increased tone are found in the proximal limb muscles, although the disorder may affect the axial musculature, producing a resistance to passive whole-body movements.

3.2.5. Tremor

> <Item 5. Tremor>
> Repetitive, regular (4-8 Hz), and rhythmic movements observed in the oral region, fingers, extremities, and trunk. Rate principally giving greater weight to the frequency and the severity of the symptoms observed objectively, however, consider the degree of distress that the subject complains of and that of the effects on the subject's quality of life due to the symptoms, as well.
>
> 0. Absent.
>
> 1. Non-specific minimal tremor, and/or mild tremor observed intermittently in a single area.
>
> 2. Mild tremor is observed persistently in a single area. Mild tremor in two or more regions and/or moderate tremor in a single area are observed intermittently.
>
> 3. Moderate tremor is observed persistently in a single area. Moderate tremor in two or more regions and/or severe tremor in a single area are observed intermittently.
>
> 4. Severe generalized tremor, and/or whole body tremor.

Tremor is an unintentional, regular, repetitive, rhythmic movement that is consistent in time and space. Body parts involved include the tongue, jaw/chin, lips, head, face, trunk, and upper and lower limbs. Most tremors occur in the hands. Sometimes tremor is a symptom of another neurological disorder, but the most common form occurs in otherwise healthy people. Some forms of tremor are inherited and run in families, while others have no known cause. Excessive alcohol consumption or alcohol withdrawal can kill certain nerve cells, resulting in tremor, especially in the hand. Other causes include an overactive thyroid and the use of certain drugs. Tremor may occur at any age but is most common in middle-aged and older persons. 'Pill rolling' tremor, a classical parkinsonian tremor which is present at rest, can occur after several years of antipsychotic drug treatment and looks as if the patient is rolling a pill between his/her fingers and thumb.

The regularity and repetitiveness of tremor movements are defined in terms of their frequency, technically expressed as Herz (Hz), or the number of excursions or cycles per second (cps). There are 2 types of parkinsonian tremor. The first is the characteristic 'resting tremor', characterized by a high amplitude and low frequency, in the range of 3-6 Hz. This type of tremor shows itself predominantly at rest and frequently decreases with purposefully directed movement of the affected part. The second type of tremor is predominantly postural. It is characterized by a low amplitude and high frequency (8-12 Hz), appears under conditions of sustained motor activity, and attenuates in the inactive state. This type of tremor is best observed in the upper limbs and the outstretched hands. Its influence can also be detected in the patient's handwriting or in a spiral drawn by the patient. It can also be observed elsewhere, for example, in the eyelids when the eyes are closed or in the protruded tongue.

<Question 2> How do I differentiate mild cases from moderate cases?
When mild or moderate tremor (or dyskinesia) persists across multiple locations, it seems unlikely to be defined in the anchor points; how is the severity of these cases defined?

Answer 2: The anchor points are not organized so as to cover all possible pathologies. However, in the case described in this question, a rating that is 1 rank higher should be considered when a single location becomes multiple locations. Thus, if mild tremor (or dyskinesia) persists across multiple locations, then a rating of moderate should be considered. Likewise, if moderate tremor (or dyskinesia) persists across multiple locations, then a rating of severe should be considered. However, this is simply a basic approach – it is not an automatic, inflexible rule. It is neither possible nor practical to define and explain in the anchor point descriptions the different levels of severity for all of the various possible pathologies, and it would be better to consider the anchor point explanations as representing only one example out of multiple possible pathologies. If a rating needs to be given for a situation that is not described in the anchor points, consider (1) whether the tremor is occurring across multiple locations, (2) what is the level of severity of tremor at each of the locations, and (3) are these tremors persistent, then decide what level of severity of the described anchor point it best corresponds to in a comprehensive and flexible manner.

<Question 3> **How do I define 'one region' for symmetrical and asymmetric manifestations?**
When rating tremor or dyskinesia, the rater should base the severity rating on whether it is localized to a single region or ranges over multiple regions. When symptoms are observed bilaterally in both arms or in both legs, should I count the right and left arms/legs as separate regions?

Answer 3: In minor or minimal cases, the symptom may sometimes be observed in only one arm or one leg, and in such cases, the rater should count it as one region. However, above a certain level of severity, the symptom is usually observed bilaterally, and in this case the rater should regard both arms or both legs as one region in the DIEPSS evaluation. In moderate or more severe cases, tremor or dyskinesia is infrequently observed on only one side; therefore, if there is an obvious asymmetric difference, it would be sensible to consider the possibility of an alternative origin for the EPS, such as organic factors or idiopathic parkinsonism, rather than a drug-induced origin.

3.2.6. Differential Diagnosis

It is sometimes difficult to differentiate antipsychotic-induced bradykinesia from the blunted affect and reduced expression of emotion characteristic of the negative symptoms of schizophrenia. It may also be difficult to distinguish between drug-induced bradykinesia and other negative symptoms of schizophrenia, such as motor retardation or lack of spontaneity. Differentiation can, however, be achieved based on the response to the administration of anticholinergic antiparkinsonian drugs and/or to a decrease in antipsychotic dosage. The behavioral features of blunted affect include a lack of manifest emotion, but there is no underlying muscular disability which would block or decrease the ability to spontaneously express emotion. In contrast, a parkinsonian facial mask is caused by both rigidity and bradykinesia of the facial muscles, so in this case, the inhibition of emotional expression is a physical phenomenon.

Bradykinesia is a physical rather than an emotional disability, the features of which are a gradual decrease in facial expressiveness and speech: decreased smiling and blinking, and slurred speech. The reduction in blink rate and the aimlessly parted lips and open mouth are helpful in differentiating between the facial masking of parkinsonism, the retardation associated with depression and the affective flattening seen in schizophrenic patients.

The differential diagnosis of drug-induced parkinsonian tremor and essential tremor is based on the patient's history and examination, although there is significant overlap between the disorders. Essential tremor is the most common of more than 20 types of tremor. The hands are most commonly affected but the head, voice, tongue, legs and trunk may also be involved. Essential tremor in the head region may be seen as a characteristic 'affirmation' ('yes-yes') or 'negation' ('no-no') motion. Onset is most common after age 40, although symptoms may appear at any age. The parkinsonian tremor is classically seen as a 'pill-rolling' action of the hands but may also affect the jaw, lips, legs and trunk. Essential tremor occurs more often during an action, whereas parkinsonian tremor tends to occur at rest. Essential tremor is relatively symmetrical, while asymmetry is more characteristic of the parkinsonian tremor (Adler, 1999). Parkinsonian tremor is likely to be associated with other abnormalities such as reduced arm-swinging, slowness of movements and tremor of the hand while walking, micrographic (small and difficult-to-read) handwriting, hypophonic speech, drooling, a shuffling gait, a stooped posture or difficulties with balance, which do not occur in essential tremor. In essential tremor, handwriting is often large and tremulous, and described as 'sloppy' or 'shaky'. The lower lip may tremble in patients with Parkinson's disease, whereas a jaw tremor is more typical of essential tremor. If a marked tremor is noted on speaking, essential tremor is more likely. When asked to tap their fingers, patients with essential tremor do so with normal speed and wide excursions, whereas patients with Parkinson's disease are slow and have reduced excursions.

3.3. Akathisia

<Item 6. Akathisia>
Akathisia consists of subjective inner restlessness, such as awareness of the inability to remain seated, restless legs, fidgetiness, and the desire to move constantly, and of objective increased motor phenomena, such as body rocking, shifting from foot to foot, stamping in place, crossing and uncrossing legs, pacing around. Rate giving greater weight to the severity of subjective symptoms and use the increased motor phenomena as evidence to support subjective symptoms. For example, rate 0 when no awareness of inner restlessness is observed, and rate 1 when only non-specific indefinite inner restlessness is obtained, even if characteristic restless movements of akathisia are observed (pseudoakathisia). In rating akathisia, consider the presence or absence of restlessness throughout the entire examination, as well.

0. Absent.

1. Non-specific minimal inner restlessness.

2. Awareness of mild inner restlessness not always resulting in subjective distress. Characteristic increased motor phenomena of akathisia may be observed.

3. Moderate inner restlessness. Results in uncomfortable symptoms and distress. Characteristic restless movements of the legs derived from the subjective inner restlessness, such as body rocking, shifting from foot to foot and stamping in place, are observed.

4. Severe inner restlessness. Results in the inability to remain seated, or moving the legs constantly. Obviously distressing condition which may induce disturbed sleep and/or anxiety states. Subject strongly desires relief of symptoms.

Section 3. DIEPSS Individual Items

3.3.1. Clinical features

Akathisia refers to a kind of restlessness, or inability to sit still. This condition is caused by antipsychotic medication. Akathisia consists of both subjective and objective components.

The subjective component includes a feeling of inner restlessness, such as awareness of an inability to remain seated, restless legs, fidgetiness and a desire to move constantly, while the objective component includes increased motor phenomena, such as body rocking while standing or sitting, changing position, fidgeting in the chair or crossing and uncrossing the legs while sitting, shifting the weight from foot to foot or stamping in place while standing, pacing around and an inability to sit down for long periods. Patients with the severe form are unable to tolerate any position, sitting, lying or standing, for more than a few minutes.

When patients who feel restless or jittery or are unable to relax are asked to be calm and to sit comfortably in the same position for a while, some characteristic signs of the objective motor components can be observed, such as fidgeting in the chair, crossing and uncrossing the legs or rocking. Akathisia can cause patients to pace hallways, repeatedly get up and down from a chair, and experience fidgety legs. The restless sensation is usually most intense in the upper legs and trunk. Akathisia also waxes and wanes; it may become inconspicuous when the patient is busy or distracted, and worsen when the patient is left alone. Patients often describe akathisia by saying "I feel like I'm jumping out of my skin". Sometimes, however, they have trouble communicating their distress and may not mention their akathisia without being asked. They may pace rapidly up and down, a presentation referred to as tasikinesia or the marching syndrome.

Akathisia occurs in approximately 20% of acute psychiatric admissions in patients receiving antipsychotic drugs (Braude et al, 1983; Ayd, 1961). It is one of the most major problems in the field of clinical psychopharmacology because the uncomfortable feeling that this side effect produces is a frequent cause of noncompliance with antipsychotic treatment. Furthermore, if it is allowed to persist, it can produce dysphoria and sometimes lead to behavioral deterioration and even suicide. It has been suggested that patients in whom acute akathisia develops may be more likely to manifest TD in the long-run (Chouinard et al, 1979; Barnes & Braude, 1984).

<Question 4> Should I rate the severity of objective movements of akathisia in the item of dyskinesia?

Patients with akathisia, especially moderate or severe cases, often exhibit an objective increase of motor phenomena, such as body rocking, shifting from one foot to another, stamping in one place, crossing and uncrossing of the legs, or pacing around, as described in the manual. Should the degree of these objective increases in motor phenomena seen in akathisia be rated in the item of dyskinesia?

Answer 4: If these increased motor phenomena can be regarded as abnormal movements, then their severity should be rated in the item of dyskinesia. In fact, dyskinetic movements are sometimes observed simultaneously in patients with chronic akathisia. In some cases, patients showing akathisia often develop minimal or mild dyskinesia later, and as the severity of dyskinetic movements progresses, so the complaint of subjective inner restlessness gradually decreases; and finally akathisia is likely to be replaced completely with dyskinesia in some cases. However, if the movement can be considered as an increase in normal activities such as walking, then any increased state of such movements should not be rated in the item of dyskinesia.

3.3.2. Differential diagnosis

It is often difficult to differentiate akathisia from a worsening psychosis or conditions such as agitation, anxiety, insomnia, attention deficit disorder, restless leg syndrome and 'acting out' behavior (Siris, 1985; van Putten, 1975; Chouinard & Margolese, 2005). The misdiagnosis of akathisia as an exacerbation of psychotic symptoms may lead to an increase in the neuroleptic dose, resulting in worsening of the akathisia. Pharmacological strategies are helpful in the differential diagnosis: β-blockers and anticholinergic drugs will relieve the symptoms and signs of akathisia, while anxiolytic drugs will benefit anxiety. If agitation worsens with an increase in the neuroleptic dosage, a reduction and a trial of treatment for akathisia is indicated. Restless leg syndrome has strong clinical similarities to akathisia but can usually be distinguished by the subjective discomfort being confined to the legs, the absence of associated internal feelings of extreme anxiety or restlessness, symptoms being present only when the patient is reclining, and the prompt relief of symptoms by walking (Tarsy, 1992). Symptoms resembling akathisia can sometimes be observed in the opiate withdrawal syndrome. Patients treated with tricyclic antidepressants for panic disorder and agoraphobia have been noted to develop jitteriness, restlessness, trouble standing still and anxiety, which can be differentiated from akathisia in that panic and phobic conditions have been reported to respond to a phenothiazine. Chronic akathisia is sometimes difficult to distinguish from other chronic drug-induced movement disorders such as tardive dystonia and tardive dyskinesia.

3.4. Dystonia

<Item 7. Dystonia>

Dystonia is a syndrome induced by the hypertonic state of muscles, manifested by stiffness, twisting, spasms, contraction, and persistent abnormal position of muscles observed in the tongue, neck, extremities, trunk, etc. Symptoms include tongue protrusion, torticollis, retrocollis, trismus, oculogyric crisis, Pisa syndrome, etc. Rate only the abnormal degree of increased muscle tone on this item. The degree of abnormal movements resulting from dystonia should be rated in the item of dyskinesia. Rate principally giving greater weight to the frequency and the severity of symptoms observed objectively, however, consider the degree of distress that the subject complains of and that of the effects on the subject's quality of life due to the symptoms, as well. Take the concomitant symptoms into consideration in rating this item, such as the subject's complaint of difficulty in swallowing, thickness of the tongue, etc.

0. Absent.

1. Impression of minimal muscle tightness, twisting or abnormal posture.

2. Mild dystonia. Mild stiffness, twisting or spasms observed in tongue, neck, extremities, trunk, or mild oculogyric crisis. The subject does not always feel distress.

3. Moderate dystonia. Moderate stiffness, twisting, contraction or oculogyric crisis. The subject often complains of distress related to the symptoms. Prompt treatment is desirable.

4. Severe dystonia observed in trunk and/or extremities. The subject has marked difficulties with activities of daily living, such as eating and walking, due to these symptoms. Urgent treatment is indicated.

3.4.1. Clinical features

Dystonia is a syndrome of hypertonicity of the muscles, characterized by sustained, often painful, muscular spasms that produce twisting, squeezing and pulling movements. The term is used to describe an uncontrollable muscle spasm which becomes evident as a contraction of the flexor and extensor muscles, leading to an abnormal position. Acute dystonia is of sudden onset, dramatic in appearance, recurrent, associated with distress and/or pain, evidenced by forceful contractions that can only sometimes be overcome with effort, and usually requires immediate treatment. Anxiety is known to trigger these dystonic reactions. The rarer tardive forms of dystonia produce more sustained contractions and abnormal positions.

The symptoms may affect the eye (blepharospasm, oculogyration), neck (torticollis, retrocollis, head turning), jaw (spasm, clenching, bruxism, trismus), tongue (protrusion), face (grimacing), larynx (hoarseness, choked voice) and pharynx (laryngo-pharyngeal constriction), and cause bizarrely bent positions of the limbs and trunk. This condition can sometimes cause the person's eyes to roll upward (oculogyric crisis), or the head to turn to the side so that the chin points toward one shoulder. Oculogyric crisis is an acute symptom which is typical of drug-induced dystonia. Trismus, or 'lockjaw', is due to a sustained contraction of the masseter muscle caused by a central inhibitory disorder, and is often observed as the initial symptom of systemic tetanus. When evaluating trismus, lockjaw due to dystonia of the masseter muscle should be rated. Other symptoms include the foot turning in as if there is uncontrollable movement of the ankle and the toe. Contractions in the mouth and pharynx are seen in some cases; the mouth may close tight, and patients feel as if they are being choked by the pharyngeal muscle contractions.

Acute dystonic reactions usually occur in the initial phase of antipsychotic therapy, 50% within 48 hours and 90% within 5 days of exposure to an antipsychotic medication (Ayd, 1961), and appear twice as often in males than in females. They are most frequent in adolescents and young adults. The prevalence of this condition has been estimated as 2.3-11.9% in patients receiving typical antipsychotic agents (Ayd, 1961, 1983).

The tardive forms of dystonia are rare, with an approximate prevalence of 3% of patients on long-term antipsychotic treatment. Some probable risk factors for tardive dystonia are younger age, male, and the presence of tardive dyskinesia (van Harten & Kahn, 1999).

<Question 5> How do I rate the abnormal movements induced by dystonia?

The dystonia item states: 'Rate only the abnormal degree of increased muscle tone on this item. The degree of abnormal movements resulting from dystonia should be rated in the item of dyskinesia.' When the origin of an abnormal movement is obviously derived from dystonia, i.e. a hypertonic state of the muscles, should I still evaluate it as dyskinesia?

Answer 5: The symptoms of dystonia and dyskinesia are related and not independent. Dystonia is defined literally as an abnormality of muscle tone (Denny-Brown's view), while it represents a disordered brain 'engram' for a particular movement that results in a dynamic disturbance between agonistic and antagonistic muscles (Dr. David Marsden's view). In the DIEPSS, the dystonia item should be used to rate the severity of abnormal muscular tonus associated principally with movements including chorea, athetosis, and static torticollis/torticollis (abnormal positions) resulting from abnormal muscle tonicity, either with or without accompanying abnormal movement. A rating in the dyskinesia item should be given if any abnormality of movement is present, regardless of the presence/absence of dystonia (abnormal muscle tone). According to these DIEPSS definitions, if a symptom with combined abnormal muscle tone and abnormal involuntary movement is observed, the degree of tonus should be rated as dystonia and the degree of abnormal movement should be rated as dyskinesia.

3.4.2. Differential diagnosis

As dystonia typically occurs in the setting of acute psychosis (acute dystonic reactions), inexperienced clinicians often misdiagnose dystonia as the psychogenic stereotyped behavior seen in patients with the catatonic type of schizophrenia. Dystonia may also be mistaken for a hysterical reaction because it can be triggered when the person is under stress. However, dystonia and similar symptoms related to psychogenic conditions can be easily differentiated by a simple therapeutic trial: there is a dramatic response to the administration of anticholinergic agents in acute dystonic reactions.

The persistent forms of dystonia, collectively called tardive dystonia, should be differentiated from the mannerisms and abnormal postures originating from schizophrenic illness. Tardive dystonia can progress over time and may be associated or mixed with other movement disorders, most commonly with tardive dyskinesia.

3.5. Dyskinesia

> <Item 8. Dyskinesia>
> Hyperkinetic abnormal movements. Apparently purposeless, irregular, and involuntary movements observed in face (muscles of facial expression), mouth (lips and perioral area), tongue, jaw, upper extremity (arms, wrists, hands, fingers), lower extremity (legs, knees, ankles, toes) and/or trunk (neck, shoulders, hips). Choreic and athetoid movements are rated, but tremor is not included. Rate principally giving greater weight to the frequency and the severity of abnormal involuntary movements observed objectively, however, consider the degree of distress that the subject complains of and that of the effects on the subject's quality of life due to the symptoms, as well. Rate movements that occur upon activation one less than those observed spontaneously.
>
> 0. Absent.
>
> 1. Non-specific minimal abnormal involuntary movements are observed.
>   Mild abnormal involuntary movements are observed intermittently in a localized area.
>
> 2. Mild abnormal involuntary movements are observed persistently in a localized area.
>   Mild abnormal involuntary movements in two or more regions and/or moderate abnormal involuntary movements in a localized area are observed intermittently.
>
> 3. Moderate abnormal involuntary movements are observed persistently in a localized area.
>   Moderate abnormal involuntary movements in two or more regions and/or severe abnormal involuntary movements in a localized area are observed intermittently.
>
> 4. Severe abnormal involuntary movements are observed.
>   The subject has difficulty with activities of daily living due to the symptoms.

3.5.1. Clinical features

Dyskinesia describes hyperkinetic abnormal movements that are irregular, purposeless and involuntary. This condition is usually associated with the prolonged use of antipsychotic drugs; this late-onset type of dyskinesia is called tardive dyskinesia (TD). The symptoms can occur in any body region, but the most common clinical presentation of TD is the bucco-lingual masticatory syndrome.

Patients may exhibit lip-smacking, tongue movements and chewing, as well as grimacing or other movements involving the facial muscles. TD may also involve the musculature of the neck, trunk and extremities, sometimes manifesting in the form of choreo-athetoid movements. The symptoms may persist for several years, even after antipsychotic withdrawal, and often become irreversible. The prevalence of TD has been estimated at 15-20% of patients receiving long-term antipsychotic treatment (Gerlach & Casey, 1988). A number of risk factors associated with greater vulnerability to TD have been reported, which include older age, female sex, a diagnosis of affective disorder, diabetes mellitus, and the use of high doses of antipsychotic medication (American Psychiatric Association, 1997). Subtypes of TD, which are considered to have the same etiology as TD but with the manifestations of acute forms, have been rarely reported; they include tardive akathisia and tardive dystonia.

<Question 6> How do I differentiate an involuntary movement from a voluntary one?
The movement in which a patient moves his/her head and tries to stop it at a specific position is considered as a voluntary movement, not as an involuntary movement, isn't it?

Answer 6: When a patient who is exhibiting dystonia (e.g., torticollis, cervical dystonia) is asked to move his/her head and stop it at a specific position, the head often goes too far and the patient tries to move it back to its original position. The original moving of the head and the corrective movement are voluntary movements, in which the patient has unquestionably moved his/her head deliberately. However, the extent to which the head goes beyond the specified position against the patient's will is considered an 'involuntary movement within a voluntary movement', and the severity of this involuntary component is rated under the dyskinesia item. In other words, if the patient's head seems to wobble, without stopping, when he/she tries to stop it at the specified position, the portion of the movement in which the patient is trying to reach the specified position is a voluntary movement, the portion in which the specified position was exceeded is an involuntary movement, and the portion in which the patient is trying to go back to the specified position is a voluntary movement. Thus, this type of movement can be considered to be composed nearly equally of voluntary and involuntary components.

3.5.2. Differential diagnosis

Symptoms that should be differentiated from TD include catatonic movements in schizophrenia, oral movements due to poorly fitting dentures and other drug-induced movement disorders such as akathisia, tremor and 'rabbit syndrome'. Unlike catatonic movements, typical TD is a spontaneous movement that occurs while the patient is at rest and involves the oro-buccal structures and the distal extremities more than other body regions. It is increased by distraction and stress, and ameliorated by activity of the involved area, by asking the patient to suppress the movements or simply by calling attention to the motion; the patient is usually unaware of the movements. To avoid misdiagnosing oral movements due to poorly fitting dentures as TD in daily clinical practice, the physician should carefully observe any movements around the oral region after the patient has taken out his/her dentures. It may be difficult to differentiate TD from chronic akathisia in some cases. The time of onset relative to initial drug exposure, location of movements in the trunk or lower extremities, coexistence of other extrapyramidal signs and response to anticholinergic drugs are helpful pieces of information, but are not always reliable in distinguishing between these two side effects. In principle, akathisia consists primarily of subjective distress; the objective movements are secondary, and are voluntary attempts to relieve the distressing internal stimuli. In contrast, while patients with TD may also show distress, this is secondary to the involuntary movements rather than the cause (Tarsy, 1992). It is virtually impossible to distinguish between TD and spontaneous dyskinesias associated with the etiology of schizophrenia itself, which were reported before the introduction of antipsychotic drugs.

3.6. Overall Severity of Extrapyramidal Symptoms

<Item9. Overall severity>
Rate overall severity of extrapyramidal symptoms, considering the severity and the frequency of individual symptoms, the degree of distress that the subject complains of, that of the effects on the subject's activities of daily living due to the symptoms, and that of the necessity for their treatments.

0. Absent.

1. Minimal or questionable.

2. Mild. Hardly affects the subject's activities of daily living. Not always feels distress.

3. Moderate. Affects the subject's activities of daily living to some degree. Often feels distress.

4. Severe. Affects the subject's activities of daily living significantly. Strongly feels distress.

The overall severity, the 9th item in the DIEPSS, assesses the severity of the patient's current EPS state based principally on the clinician's global impression of how EPS are affecting the subject's activities of daily living and on how strongly distressed the patient feels. It corresponds to the 'Severity of Illness' in the Clinical Global Impressions (CGI) Scale (Guy 1976), as the 8 individual items for EPS in the DIEPSS correspond to the 30 items for psychotic symptoms in the Positive and Negative Syndrome Scale (PANSS). Although the overall severity item in the DIEPSS is graded in 5 levels, from '0 (normal)' to '4 (severe)', it is analyzed independently from 8 individual items; using this approach has enabled the different EPS severity profiles of typical and atypical antipsychotics to be distinguished in some clinical trials.

4. Reliability of the DIEPSS

The DIEPSS has been confirmed to have a high level of reliability by both the inter-rater reliability test and the test-retest reliability test.

4.1. Inter-rater Reliability

4.1.1. Japanese study

The following procedure was followed to establish the inter-rater reliability of the DIEPSS (Inada, 1996). A total of 6 psychiatrists participated in the study. They were divided into 3 pairs: each pair used the DIEPSS to rate the extrapyramidal symptoms observed in psychiatric patients on antipsychotic treatment in a jointly conducted assessment interview. Before the initiation of the study, extensive training for rating EPS with the DIEPSS was given to the 2 psychiatrists in pair 1, whereas deliberately inadequate training was given to the psychiatrists in pairs 2 and 3, although these raters were specialist psychiatrists with more than 5 years of experience. The distribution of psychiatric diagnoses and the number of subjects enrolled in the study are shown in **Table 1**. Most of the subjects rated by pair 1 and pair 2 were schizophrenic patients, while elderly patients with dementia were selected as subjects for pair 3.

Table 1. Distribution of Psychiatric Diagnoses (Inada, 1996)

Diagnosis (ICD-10)	Pair 1 (n=21)	Pair 2 (n=26)	Pair 3 (n=17)
Schizophrenia (F20)	18	22	0
Bipolar Affective Disorder (F31)	2	1	0
Mild Mental Retardation (F70)	0	2	0
Dementia in Alzheimer's Disease (F00)	0	0	14
Dementia in Other Diseases Classified elsewhere (F02)	0	0	2
Others	1	1	1

For 4 of the items (item 3, sialorrhea, item 5, tremor; item 6, akathisia; item 8, dyskinesia), there were not many severe cases and no moderate-to-severe cases among the enrolled patients. Therefore, previously recorded videos of 6 patients with severe symptoms (2 with sialorrhea, 1 with tremor, 1 with akathisia and 2 with dyskinesia) and 6 patients with moderate-to-severe symptoms (2 with sialorrhea, 1 with tremor, 1 with akathisia and 2 with dyskinesia) were played when all 6 raters were in attendance, and each pair independently rated each item on the videotape in addition to their live patients.

Table 2 presents the calculations of the percentage concordance (agreement) rate, the percentage consistency rate between the 2 evaluation sessions (the percentage concordance rate was calculated on the basis that when the difference in the score between two raters was ±1 point, the ratings were judged to be consistent), the concordance rate calculated by Cohen's kappa coefficient and the Analysis of Variance Intraclass Correlation Coefficient (ANOVA ICC) (Giraudeau & Mary, 2001). for each of the 9 DIEPSS items and each pair of raters.

Table 2. Results of inter-rater reliability test for DIEPSS (Inada, 1996)

DIEPSS 8 items	Evaluator pair (N)	Concordance rate (%)	Back and forth Concordance rate (%)	Cohen's κ	ANOVA ICC
1. Gait	Pair 1 (N=21)	85.7	100	0.809	0.942
	Pair 2 (N=26)	57.7	96.2	0.389	0.631
	Pair 3 (N=17)	88.2	100	0.850	0.972
2. Bradykinesia	Pair 1 (N=21)	71.4	100	0.617	0.894
	Pair 2 (N=26)	34.6	96.2	0.045	0.506
	Pair 3 (N=17)	58.8	94.1	0.476	0.811
3. Sialorrhea	Pair 1 (N=23)	95.7	100	0.883	0.983
	Pair 2 (N=28)	85.7	100	0.651	0.915
	Pair 3 (N=19)	68.4	100	0.387	0.792
4. Muscle rigidity	Pair 1 (N=21)	76.2	100	0.593	0.894
	Pair 2 (N=26)	69.2	96.2	0.494	0.813
	Pair 3 (N=17)	58.8	94.1	0.396	0.802
5. Tremor	Pair 1 (N=22)	77.3	100	0.667	0.924
	Pair 2 (N=27)	66.7	100	0.514	0.822
	Pair 3 (N=18)	61.1	88.9	0.452	0.607
6. Akathisia	Pair 1 (N=22)	86.4	100	0.697	0.945
	Pair 2 (N=27)	88.9	100	0.822	0.959
	Pair 3 (N=18)	72.2	94.4	0.458	0.737
7. Dystonia	Pair 1 (N=21)	95.2	100	0.921	0.987
	Pair 2 (N=26)	88.5	92.3	0.533	0.633
	Pair 3 (N=17)	76.5	94.1	0.460	0.828
8. Dyskinesia	Pair 1 (N=23)	85.7	100	0.692	0.943
	Pair 2 (N=28)	82.1	96.4	0.440	0.827
	Pair 3 (N=19)	68.4	94.7	0.301	0.793
9. Overall severity	Pair 1 (N=21)	76.2	100	0.685	0.908
	Pair 2 (N=26)	69.2	100	0.419	0.574
	Pair 3 (N=17)	64.7	94.1	0.521	0.776

Relatively low values for the percentage concordance rate and Cohen's kappa coefficient were observed for 2 items, gait and bradykinesia, for pair 2, who had not had sufficient visual training before using the DIEPSS. For the other items, the evaluations performed by all 3 pairs of psychiatrists was generally stable and showed good agreement with each other. On the whole, the concordance rates were high; in particular, pair 1, who had extensive training, showed extremely high concordance rates for all the items. This indicates that proper rater training is essential in order to achieve good inter-rater agreement, as reported by Gerlach et al (1993). Furthermore, reliance on only the literature provided in the manual for training equips raters with insufficient ability to perform precise evaluations of the severity of movement disorders; visual recognition, as provided by the training videos, is an important aspect. Rater pair 3, who investigated various forms of dementia, also showed high concordance rates, thereby indicating that the DIEPSS is a very useful scale with a high level of reliability not only for psychiatric diseases centering around schizophrenia but also for patients with dementia who are taking antipsychotic drugs.

The results demonstrate the high reliability of this scale and also indicate that the selection of subjects for this reliability study was valid: the severity of the cases chosen for each item of the DIEPSS

Section 4. Reliability of the DIEPSS

was widely distributed from 0 (normal) to 4 (severe).

4.1.2. Korean study

In the Korean inter-rater reliability study, the metric properties of the DIEPSS were assessed using three independent samples of subjects. Inter-rater reliability was evaluated using 40 subjects. Two adequately trained raters independently assessed each patient using the DIEPSS. Both were blind to the assessment of the other rater and to the medication regimen and dosage. The inter-rater reliability was examined using intraclass correlation coefficients (ICCs). Agreement in the inter-rater reliability of the individual items was high, with ICCs ranging from 0.76 to 0.96, suggesting that the item definitions and the scoring method of the DIEPSS are adequate and clear. The ICC for the total score of the DIEPSS was 0.97, showing a high level of reliability.

4.2. Test-retest Reliability

In judging test-retest reliability, it is important to note that it is impossible to provide identical subjects for each set of raters unless video recorded cases are used. However, when video rating is used with the DIEPSS, the item of muscle rigidity cannot be rated, since this rating requires a physical examination. Hence, it is best to select patients who have had no major change in their EPS between the rating sessions. As a logical consequence, because a serious symptom cannot be left untreated for 3 weeks, the subjects should be limited to those with relatively mild EPS. If there is still a difference in rating, a difficult situation arises in which it is practically impossible to tell whether the difference is due to a problem with the scale (i.e. the scale has no test-retest reliability), a problem with the rater (e.g. an inability to produce stable ratings due to a lack of training), or whether a chance symptom occurred at only one of the rating sessions, and there are no problems with either the scale or the rater.

4.2.1. Japanese study

The study of test-retest reliability was performed by a trained psychiatrist (Inada, 1996). Using the DIEPSS, the rater evaluated extrapyramidal symptoms in 34 male chronic schizophrenic patients (age range: 37-72 years) on 2 separate occasions, with an interval of more than 3 weeks. The patients' psychiatric symptoms had remained stable, and they had been receiving steady doses of the same maintenance antipsychotic drug, for more than 1 year. Patients whose psychiatric symptoms changed sufficiently to warrant a change in their treatment were excluded. The concordance rates and Cohen's kappa values for the 9 DIEPSS items are shown in **Table 3**. With this study design, it is difficult to confirm whether the level of disagreement between the 2 evaluations derives from problems with the scale itself or from detecting real changes in symptoms. Taking this situation into consideration, the Cohen's kappa values observed here, ranging from 0.461 to 0.747, can be considered acceptable.

Table 3. Results of test-retest reliability test for DIEPSS (Inada, 1996)

DIEPSS 8 items	Concordance rate (%)	Cohen's κ
1. Gait	64.7	0.508
2. Bradykinesia	61.7	0.461
3. Sialorrhea	73.5	0.598
4. Muscle rigidity	70.6	0.532
5. Tremor	76.5	0.573
6. Akathisia	73.5	0.624
7. Dystonia	79.4	0.653
8. Dyskinesia	82.4	0.747
9. Overall severity	76.5	0.646

4.2.2. Korean study

In the Korean test–retest reliability study (Kim et al, 2002a), DIEPSS scores were evaluated twice, with a 2-week-interval, in 42 patients who had been on steady maintenance antipsychotic treatment for at least 4 weeks. No change in the antipsychotic dose or adjunctive medication was allowed until the second examination had been completed. All of the items showed adequate reliability, with ICCs ranging from 0.60 to 0.91, suggesting stability of the rating across time. Regarding the individual items, the ICCs for the tremor and bradykinesia items were somewhat lower than those for the other items in this study. This may have resulted from short-term variations or the evolution of these symptoms (Barnes & Kane, 1994; Owens, 1999). It is also possible that they could have been affected by modifying factors such as diurnal variation or anxiety (Owens, 1999). There is also the possibility of variation in rating performance over time. In assessing test–retest reliability, repeated evaluations using video recordings may have offered an advantage over the live evaluation method (Gerlach et al, 1993), except when assessing the regional manifestations of rigidity.

4.3. Training Utilities

In order to establish extremely high inter-rater reliability, DIEPSS workshops have been held since September 2001 in Japan. These use video clips showing representative, standardized examples of symptom severity for each of the anchor points in each of the DIEPSS items. The DIEPSS has begun to be used in clinical practice in various psychiatric centers in Japan; by April 2009, a total of 105 workshops had been conducted nationwide, and nearly 2,300 Japanese psychiatrists and pharmacists had received rating training. In 2007, DIEPSS workshops were started outside Japan, in countries including Korea, China, Taiwan and the United States. In parallel with this expansion, the training DVD of the original English version, which presents the contents of the DIEPSS workshops, was completed. Extremely high concordance rates have been demonstrated among raters who received training at these workshops before starting work on clinical trials.

5. Validity of the DIEPSS

5.1. Factor Structure

Corroboration of the factor structure is important in verifying the construct validity of a rating instrument (Martinez-Martin et al, 1994). If the factor structure of the DIEPSS is confirmed in future studies, the individual factor scores may be useful in clinical research and clinical trials in schizophrenic patients receiving antipsychotic treatment. Assessment of the factor structure using a principal component factor analysis has been conducted independently in Japan and Korea. In both studies, 4 factors were identified, suggesting that the DIEPSS has multidimensional characteristics. The modest degree of correlation among these factors implies that they reflect different aspects of drug-induced EPS. These results suggest that the DIEPSS is a valid multidimensional rating scale that can evaluate distinct dimensions of EPS, and that it has an advantage in allowing the comprehensive assessment of drug-induced EPS. As shown by the summaries of the detailed results of the 2 studies below, the results are consistent with previous reports of a strong correlation between the hyperkinetic forms of drug-induced EPS (Muscettola et al, 1999; van Harten et al, 1997).

5.1.1. Japanese study

The DIEPSS was assessed in 206 psychiatric patients who showed some degree of EPS while receiving antipsychotic drugs (Inada, 1996). The subjects included 142 males and 64 females, with a mean age of 55 years; the most common psychiatric diagnosis was schizophrenia (190 patients), followed by schizoaffective disorder (10 patients) and affective disorder (6 patients). A Varimax rotation was conducted after principal component analysis had been performed using the data from the 8 individual items of the DIEPSS in these subjects. **Table 4** shows the resultant rotated factor structure. Three items were extracted as the first factors: gait, bradykinesia and muscle rigidity (percentage of variance: 27%), and two items were extracted as the second factors: sialorrhea and tremor (percentage of variance: 16%). Both the first and the second factors are items related to parkinsonism, and 43% of the distributions of the DIEPSS were explained by these 5 items. The third factors were akathisia and dystonia (percentage of variance: 13%), which were considered to be rating items related to acute EPS other than parkinsonism. The fourth and last factor was dyskinesia, which represented late-onset extrapyramidal symptoms including tardive dyskinesia (percentage of variance: 12%). These 4 factors account for 68% of the variance of the DIEPSS.

Table 4. Factor structure of the 8 individual items of the DIEPSS (Inada, 1996)

DIEPSS 8 items	1 (27%)	2 (16%)	3 (13%)	4 (12%)
1. Gait	**0.87**			
2. Bradykinesia	**0.81**	0.25		0.27
3. Sialorrhea		**0.79**		0.28
4. Muscle rigidity	**0.62**			
5. Tremor		**0.85**		
6. Akathisia			**0.83**	
7. Dystonia	0.22		**0.59**	
8. Dyskinesia				**0.94**

Factor loadings of 0.5 or more are shown in bold; factor loadings of 0.2 or less are not shown.

5.1.2. Korean study

The factor structure was assessed using a principal component factor analysis with an oblique rotation (Hair et al, 1998) in 100 Korean subjects (Kim et al., 2002a). The factor analysis identified 4 factors, which accounted for 80.4% of the total variance. The items extracted as the first factor were gait, bradykinesia and rigidity, which accounted for 28.8% of the total variance. The items extracted as the second factor were sialorrhea and tremor, which accounted for 19.3% of the total variance. The items extracted as the third factor were dystonia and dyskinesia, accounting for 17.6% of the total variance. The fourth factor was akathisia, accounting for 14.8% of the total variance. Spearman correlation analyses showed a modest degree of correlation among the factors, with correlation coefficients ranging from 0.22 (P=0.03; between Factor 3 and Factor 4) to 0.37 (P < 0.001; between Factor 1 and Factor 2). There was no significant correlation between Factor 2 and Factor 4 (Spearman's r= 0.13, P=0.21). Factors 1 and 2 are related to hypokinetic and non-hypokinetic parkinsonism, respectively. Dystonia and dyskinesia were clustered together as Factor 3; this factor relates to tardive syndrome, since all 8 patients with dystonia in this Korean study satisfied the criteria for tardive dystonia, as proposed by Burke et al (1982). Factor 4 is an independent factor involving only akathisia.

5.2. Concurrent Validity

5.2.1. Correlation between the DIEPSS and other EPS scales

The concurrent validity of the DIEPSS was examined using the Simpson-Angus Scale (SAS), the Barnes Akathisia Scale (BAS) and the Abnormal Involuntary Movement Scale (AIMS) as external validation scales (Inada, 1996). The correlations between these scales are shown in **Table 5**. Items 1 to 5 in the DIEPSS cover the symptoms of parkinsonism. When the concurrent validity of the DIEPSS and the SAS was investigated in 21 male schizophrenic patients (age range: 36–68 yrs) on maintenance therapy with an antipsychotic drug, the correlation coefficient of the total scores for the 8 individual items of the DIEPSS and the total score in the SAS was 0.82; however, when only the first 5 items of the DIEPSS (which relate to parkinsonism and correspond to the whole of the SAS) were included in the comparison, a very high correlation of 0.93 was confirmed. On the other hand, the correlation coefficient of the overall rating in the DIEPSS and the total score in the SAS was somewhat low, at 0.64. In addition, the correlation between the severity of akathisia (Item 6) in the DIEPSS and the overall severity (global clinical assessment) in the BAS was high (r=0.97), as was the correlation between the severity of dyskinesia (Item 8) in the DIEPSS and item 8 (severity of abnormal movement) in the AIMS (r=0.96).

Table 5. Concurrent validity of DIEPSS with other EPS scales (Inada, 1996)

External standard	DIEPSS items	Number of patients	Correlation coefficient
Simpson-Angus Scale	Subtotal (Items 1-5)	21	0.93
	Subtotal (Items 1-8)	21	0.82
	Item 9	21	0.64
Barnes Akathisia Scale	Item 6	18	0.97
Abnormal Involuntary Movement Scale	Item 8	28	0.96

Section 5. Validity of the DIEPSS

To assess the concurrent validity in the Korean study, a total of 100 subjects were evaluated to determine whether other EPS scales (SAS, BAS and AIMS) correlated with the corresponding items in the DIEPSS using the Spearman rank correlation test. The DIEPSS scores showed strongly significant correlations with those obtained from the SAS, BAS and AIMS, with Spearman rank correlation coefficients ranging from 0.88 to 0.97 ($P < 0.001$). The results of both the Japanese and Korean studies clearly support the capacity of the DIEPSS to assess drug-induced parkinsonism (Items 1-5), akathisia (Item 6) and dyskinesia (Item 8).

5.2.2. Comparison with western scales in a double-blind study of olanzapine

The superiority of olanzapine to haloperidol with respect to a decreased incidence of treatment-emergent EPS in patients with schizophrenia has been demonstrated in studies conducted in Japan and western countries. The patients in the western trials were primarily Caucasian. The EPS measurements used in the western trials included the SAS, the BAS and the AIMS, while the DIEPSS was used in Japan. In order to clarify how the DIEPSS captures EPS profiles, we retrospectively compared the baseline prevalence and treatment-emergent incidence of EPS in the Japanese and western trials. Specifically, the prevalence and incidence of dyskinesia, akathisia and parkinsonism were compared between the Japanese trial and an international trial to determine whether appropriate definitions can be derived using the DIEPSS, assuming that comparable prevalence and incidence rates for the syndromes would be observed when any differences in residual antipsychotic exposure at the initiation of study treatment were accounted for. For the incidence of all EPS syndromes, odds ratios were similar between the two studies, indicating that appropriate criteria for the clinical diagnosis of these EPS syndromes could be established based on the DIEPSS. This study suggests that the DIEPSS can be used operationally to define the presence or absence, and make a clinical diagnosis, of specific EPS syndromes (Inada et al, 2003).

5.3. Evaluation of Optimal Cut-Off Scores

Optimal cut-off scores were determined for the DIEPSS in comparison with other widely used rating scales. In evaluating the incidence and/or prevalence of EPS using the DIEPSS, a severity score of 2 or more in the relevant DIEPSS individual items is considered diagnostic of the symptoms defined by the items. For akathisia to be diagnosed, the dystonia and dyskinesia scores should be ≥2. For the categorical diagnosis of parkinsonism, the score must be ≥3 on one item or ≥2 on two items among the five DIEPSS items of gait, bradykinesia, sialorrhea, muscle rigidity and tremor.

The evaluation of the optimal cut-off score using receiver operating characteristic (ROC) analysis has been reported in previous studies on akathisia and tardive dyskinesia (Sacdev & Kruk, 1994; Cassady et al, 1997). For the SAS, drug-induced parkinsonism was diagnosed if the total SAS score was 4 or more (Simpson & Angus, 1970). For the BAS, akathisia was diagnosed if the score on the global assessment item was 2 or more (Barnes, 1989). Tardive dyskinesia was diagnosed by the Research Diagnostic Criteria for Tardive Dyskinesia (RDC TD) using AIMS (Schooler & Kane, 1982).

The optimal cut-off scores for drug-induced parkinsonism, akathisia and tardive dyskinesia in the DIEPSS were examined using ROC analysis (Murphy et al, 1987) in 100 Korean subjects (Kim et al, 2002a). The assessment of drug-induced parkinsonism by the DIEPSS was made by obtaining the sum of the scores for the 5 individual items gait, bradykinesia, sialorrhea, rigidity and tremor. Akathisia and tardive dyskinesia were represented by the scores for Item 6 and Item 8, respectively. ROC analysis showed that a total score of 5 for the five items covering parkinsonism in the DIEPSS was the optimal cut-off score for drug-induced parkinsonism (sensitivity, 0.89; specificity, 0.92). Thus, a total score of 5 or more for these five items in the DIEPSS indicates the presence of parkinsonism.

With regard to a definite diagnosis of drug-induced parkinsonism, this can be made when there are three or more items with a severity rating of mild among the five DIEPSS items for parkinsonism. The optimal cut-off score for akathisia in the DIEPSS was 2 (sensitivity, 1.00; specificity, 0.96). A DIEPSS akathisia score of 2 (awareness of mild inner restlessness not always resulting in subjective distress) is identical with the criterion for drug-induced akathisia defined by the BAS (Barnes, 1989), and is also in line with the criterion for the diagnosis of akathisia proposed by Sachdev and Kruk (1994). The optimal cut-off score for tardive dyskinesia in the DIEPSS was 2 (sensitivity, 0.94; specificity, 0.87). A DIEPSS tardive dyskinesia score of 2 (mild severity in 2 or more regions or moderate severity intermittently observed in a localized area) is generally consistent with the RDC TD criteria (Schooler & Kane, 1982), which require a rating of mild in at least 2 regions or a moderate rating in at least one region.

5.4. Predictive Validity

The predictive validity of the DIEPSS was examined in a study of the concomitant use of antiparkinsonian drugs with antipsychotics (Inada, 1996). In this study, an antiparkinsonian drug, biperiden (3-6 mg/day), was administered for 1 week to 7 male schizophrenic patients (age range: 34-64 yrs) who developed some form of EPS during typical antipsychotic therapy. **Figure 2** shows the time-course of changes in the total scores for the 8 individual items of the DIEPSS before and after the administration of biperiden. The patients initially complained of EPS severe enough to require treatment with an antiparkinsonian drug (a total of 6-13 points for the 8 individual items of the DIEPSS in this investigation). After 1 week of concomitant use of the antiparkinsonian drug, the EPS symptoms gradually diminished, and a significant reduction was observed in the total scores for the 8 individual items of the DIEPSS compared to baseline (before treatment) ($P < 0.05$; Wilcoxon signed rank test).

Section 5. Validity of the DIEPSS

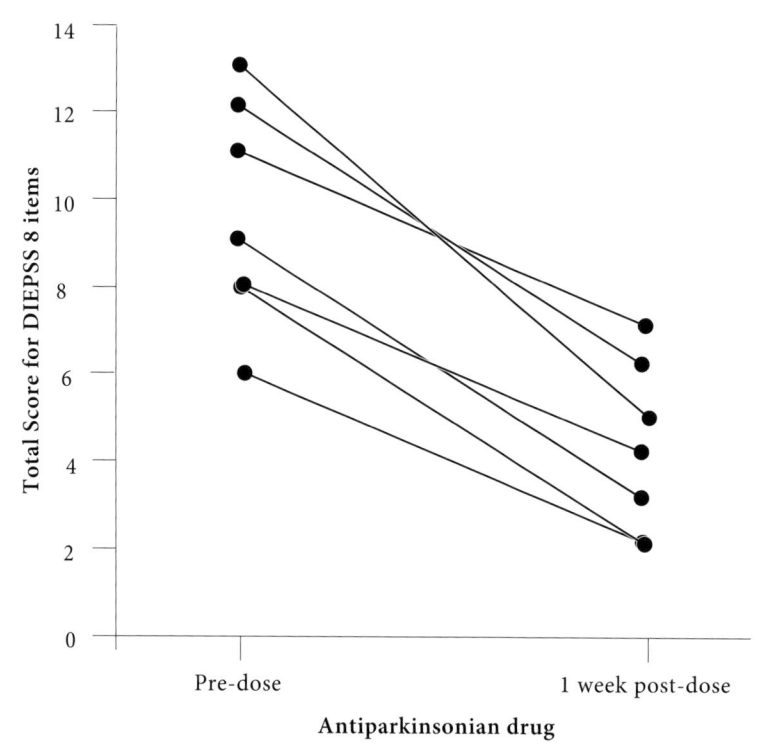

Figure 2. Time course of changes in the total scores for the 8 individual items of the DIEPSS during the administration of an antiparkinsonian drug. (Inada, 1996)

As detailed in the next chapter, a number of double-blind clinical trials comparing the efficacy and tolerability of typical and atypical antipsychotic drugs in the treatment of schizophrenia have been conducted in Japan using the DIEPSS as the rating scale. These results also help to estimate the predicted number of subjects needed to elicit a true picture of the different EPS profiles of typical and atypical antipsychotics.

6. Clinical application of the DIEPSS

6.1. Comparison of EPS profiles between typical and atypical antipsychotics

Since 1997, second-generation antipsychotic drugs, which have been shown to have a lower frequency of EPS than conventional typical antipsychotic drugs such as haloperidol, have been developed in Japan. Favorable EPS profiles have been shown for second generation antipsychotic agents such as olanzapine (Inada et al, 2002, 2003), quetiapine (Inada, 2002;), aripiprazole, blonanserin (Inada et al, 2008), risperidone depot, sertindole, ziprasidone, paliperidone, lurasidone, clozapine and others in phase III clinical trials which have used the DIEPSS to rate the severity of EPS. In addition, in a comparative study of olanzapine and fluphenazine in post-traumatic stress disorder (PTSD) patients conducted in Croatia in 2004, ratings obtained with the DIEPSS showed that olanzapine, an atypical antipsychotic drug, produced a significantly lower frequency of EPS compared to fluphenazine, a typical antipsychotic drug (Pivac et al, 2004). Virtually all double-blind clinical studies comparing atypical and typical antipsychotic drugs conducted in Japan using the DIEPSS have demonstrated that atypical antipsychotics have a significantly superior EPS profile compared to typical antipsychotics. Some of these data are summarized in this chapter.

6.1.1. Comparison of EPS profiles between olanzapine and haloperidol

Previous clinical trials have clearly shown the superiority of olanzapine over haloperidol with regard to the EPS profile in schizophrenic patients. Inada et al. (2002) reported a difference in the EPS profiles between olanzapine and haloperidol in a double-blind comparative study designed to examine the safety and efficacy of both drugs in the treatment of schizophrenia in Japan (Ishigooka et al., 2001). The DIEPSS was used to evaluate 182 patients enrolled in this 8-week study. The primary safety analysis was the maximum change (which could be either a decrease or an increase) from baseline in the DIEPSS total score. Secondary analyses included the size of the change from baseline to the maximum DIEPSS total score, the change from baseline to endpoint (LOCF) in the DIEPSS total score, and the rank sum of the maximum change (which could be either a decrease or an increase) from baseline in the individual items of the DIEPSS. The incidence of treatment-emergent extrapyramidal adverse events was also analyzed using the DIEPSS (**Figure 3**). The olanzapine group showed statistically significant superiority to the haloperidol group in the primary analysis (P<0.001). The secondary analyses also demonstrated olanzapine's superiority with regard to the total, parkinsonism, akathisia and overall severity scores (all P≤0.014). Categorical analysis of treatment-emergent akathisia and parkinsonian syndromes at the endpoint showed improvement in the olanzapine group but worsening in the haloperidol group. The results from this study suggest that, as in Caucasian populations, olanzapine is a safe treatment in Japanese patients who are chronically ill with schizophrenia.

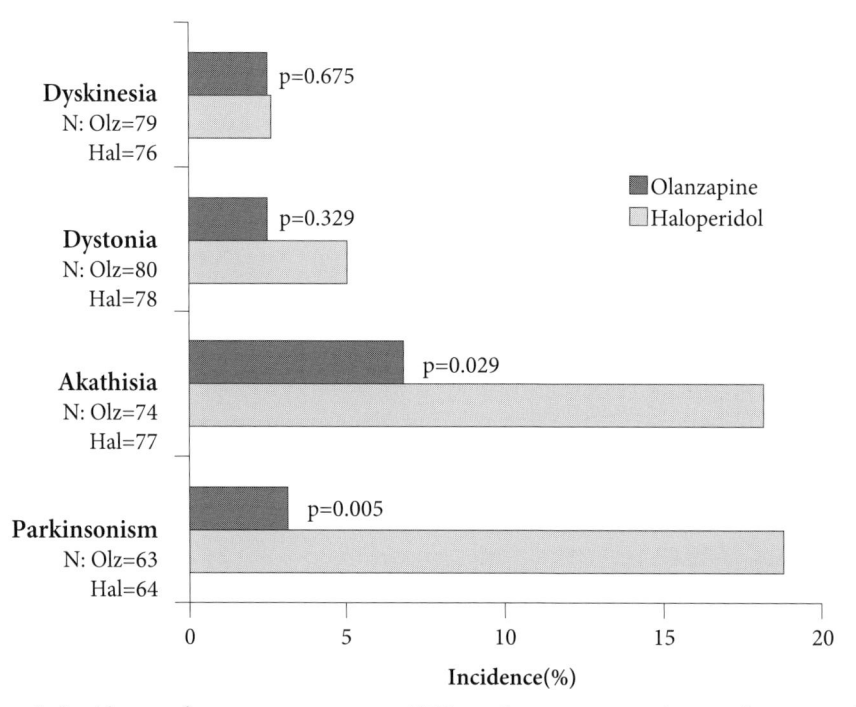

Figure 3. Incidence of treatment-emergent EPS syndromes at any time as determined by DIEPSS.

6.1.2. Comparison of EPS profiles between olanzapine and fluphenazine

Combat-related PTSD is often complicated by other psychiatric comorbidities and refractory to treatment. Pivac et al. (2004) performed an open, comparative 6-week study comparing olanzapine (n=28) with fluphenazine (n=27), at doses in the range of 5-10 mg/day, as monotherapy for 55 male patients with psychotic combat-related PTSD. EPS were evaluated using the DIEPSS. After 3 and 6 weeks of treatment, olanzapine was significantly more efficacious than fluphenazine in reducing symptoms on the PANSS (negative, general psychopathology subscale, supplementary items) and Watson's PTSD (avoidance, increased arousal) subscales, while both treatments had a similar effect on the symptoms listed in the PANSS positive and Watson's trauma re-experiencing subscales. Fluphenazine induced more extrapyramidal symptoms. Prolongation of the treatment for 3 additional weeks did not affect the efficacy of either drug. The authors concluded that although both fluphenazine and olanzapine were effective for the particular symptom profile of psychotic combat-related PTSD, olanzapine was better than fluphenazine in reducing most of the psychotic and PTSD symptoms, and was better tolerated in psychotic PTSD patients.

6.1.3. Comparison of EPS profiles between quetiapine and haloperidol

Quetiapine fumarate is known to have a superior EPS profile compared to first-generation antipsychotics in the treatment of schizophrenia. Indeed, quetiapine fumarate has been placed second to clozapine as the recommended antipsychotic agent that is least likely to cause EPS in the US Expert Consensus Guideline Series: Treatment of Schizophrenia ([No authors listed], 1999). Inada (2002) reported the favorable EPS profile of quetiapine fumarate compared to haloperidol in a double-blind trial in the treatment of schizophrenia conducted in Japan.

A total of 197 schizophrenic subjects were enrolled in this 8-week study. EPS were evaluated using the DIEPSS at baseline and at 1, 2, 3, 4, 6 and 8 weeks after starting either quetiapine fumarate (n=100) or haloperidol (n=97) or until discontinuation. Patients whose DIEPSS was evaluated at both a baseline and another postbaseline point were included in the analyses. The mean (± SD) values for the quetiapine fumarate-treated patients with regard to the mean dose and the maximum dose were 226.3±122.2 and 315.3±182.0 mg/day, respectively. The corresponding values for the haloperidol-treated patients were 6.7±3.6 and 9.6±5.1mg/day, respectively.

Significantly fewer (P<0.001) quetiapine fumarate-treated patients (30.0%) than haloperidol-treated patients (56.7%) required antiparkinsonian medication during study participation. The concomitant use rates of antiparkinsonian agents at 8 weeks after starting treatment were 25% for the quetiapine fumarate group and 60% for the haloperidol group, and the concomitant use volumes (biperiden equivalents) were 0.9±1.8mg/day for the quetiapine fumarate group and 2.8±3.4mg/day for the haloperidol group, showing significantly lower use rates and volumes in the quetiapine fumarate group (P<0.001, P=0.013).

The number of patients who did not complete treatment was 34 in the quetiapine fumarate group and 43 in the haloperidol group, the difference being non-significant. There was, however, a significant difference between the two groups regarding the reasons for discontinuation (P>0.001). The patients in the quetiapine fumarate group were inclined to be withdrawn due to aggravation of symptoms, whereas those in the haloperidol group were more likely to be withdrawn due to adverse drug reactions.

The quetiapine fumarate group showed statistically significant improvement over the haloperidol group (P<0.001) with regard to the maximum change from baseline in the total DIEPSS score (P<0.001), the overall severity score (P<0.001) and the akathisia (P=0.011), dystonia (P=0.012), dyskinesia (P=0.034) and parkinsonian subscale scores (P<0.001). The within-group DIEPSS total score was significantly improved (P=0.003) for the quetiapine fumarate-treated patients but significantly worsened (P<0.001) for the haloperidol-treated patients. The total DIEPSS score, parkinsonian subscale score and the overall severity item score were also significantly (P<0.001) improved for the endpoint change (LOCF) in the quetiapine fumarate-treated patients compared to the haloperidol-treated patients. For the incidence of treatment-emergent EPS syndromes determined by the DIEPSS at any time, the incidence of parkinsonism, akathisia, dystonia and dyskinesia was significantly higher in the haloperidol group than in the quetiapine fumarate group (**Figure 4**). For the incidence of treatment-emergent EPS determined by the DIEPSS at the endpoint, a significantly higher incidence was observed in the haloperidol group than that in the quetiapine fumarate group in the dyskinesia item (P=0.012) and the parkinsonian subscale score (P=0.037).

These results are similar to those obtained in double-blind comparisons of quetiapine and haloperidol conducted in the US. Thus, the favorable EPS profile of quetiapine fumarate has been demonstrated using the DIEPSS.

Section 6. Clinical application of the DIEPSS

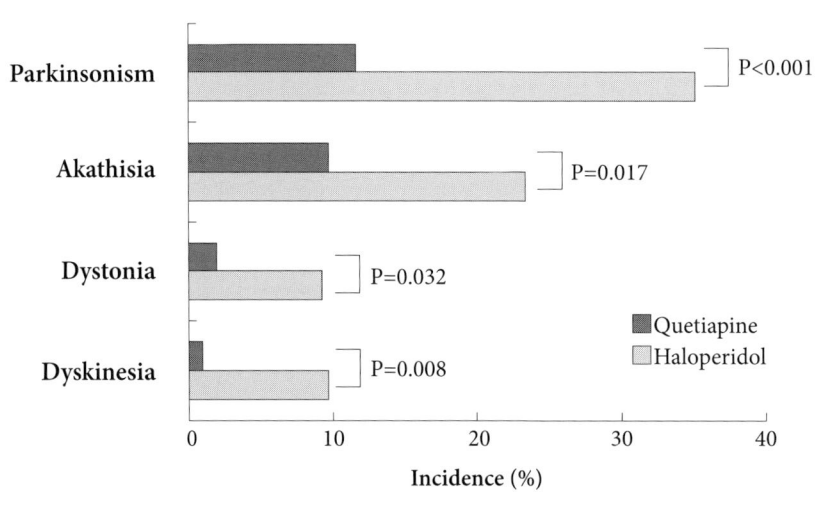

Figure 4. Incidence of treatment-emergent EPS symptoms at any time as determined by DIEPSS.

6.1.4. Comparison of EPS profiles between aripiprazole and haloperidol

Aripiprazole, a partial agonist at members of the D2 subfamily of dopamine receptors, has been reported to have a more favorable EPS profile than haloperidol in double-blind clinical studies conducted in the US (Kane et al, 2002). These EPS profiles have also been confirmed in a Japanese 8-week randomized, double-blind clinical study, which compared the safety and efficacy of aripiprazole and haloperidol in a total of 240 schizophrenic patients using the DIEPSS.

Changes from baseline to maximum in the DIEPSS scores were significantly smaller in the aripiprazole group than in the haloperidol group for the overall severity score (P=0.0003), the 5 items of the parkinsonian score (P=0.0000) and the DIEPSS total score (P=0.0001), while no significant differences were observed in akathisia (P=0.2981), dystonia (P=0.1347) or dyskinesia (P=0.7442).

Changes from baseline to endpoint were also significantly smaller in the aripiprazole-treated patients than in the haloperidol-treated patients for the overall severity score (P=0.0094), the 5 items of the parkinsonian score (P=0.0049) and the DIEPSS total score (P=0.0187) (Table 6).

The occurrence rate of treatment-emergent symptoms (DIEPSS individual item scores ≥1) was significantly higher in haloperidol-treated patients than in aripiprazole-treated patients with regard to the DIEPSS items of gait (P=0.0432), bradykinesia (P=0.0503), sialorrhea (P=0.0036), muscle rigidity (P=0.0153), tremor (P=0.0114) and akathisia (P=0.0399). The number of patients with at least 1 adverse event, as indicated by a change in at least 1 DIEPSS individual item, was also significantly higher in the haloperidol group than in the aripiprazole group (P=0.0003).

The incidence of treatment-emergent EPS determined by the DIEPSS at any time was significantly higher in the haloperidol group than in the aripiprazole group for the 5 parkinsonian items (haloperidol n=28, 27.7% vs. aripiprazole n=10, 10.4%; P=0.002) and akathisia (haloperidol n=29, 25.4% vs. aripiprazole n=16, 15.8%; P=0.019). The incidence of treatment-emergent parkinsonism at the endpoint as assessed by the DIEPSS was significantly higher (P=0.010) in the haloperidol-treated patients (n=15, 14.9%) than in the aripiprazole-treated patients (n=4, 4.2%).

Based on these results, the DIEPSS was capable of distinguishing between the EPS profiles of aripiprazole and haloperidol, and the more favorable EPS profile of aripiprazole compared to haloperidol was thus confirmed in the Japanese double-blind comparative study.

Section 6. Clinical application of the DIEPSS

Table 6. Change from baseline to endpoint (LOCF) in DIEPSS total score

DIEPSS Score	Therapy	N	Baseline		Endpoint			Change		Within Group p-Value[1]	Therapy p-Value[2]
			Mean	SD	Mean	SD	Median	Mean	SD		
Total	Arp	119	3.3	4.4	3.34	4.24	0	0.04	3.72	0.8604	0.0187
	Hal	119	2.98	3.78	4.25	4.48	0	1.27	4.13	0.0005	
Parkinsonism	Arp	119	2.19	3.02	2.03	2.82	0	-0.16	2.12	0.1111	0.0049
	Hal	119	1.97	2.64	2.68	3.12	0	0.71	2.71	0.002	
Akathisia	Arp	120	0.14	0.55	0.28	0.77	0	0.14	0.83	0.0545	0.6742
	Hal	119	0.17	0.51	0.31	0.72	0	0.14	0.78	0.0437	
Dystonia	Arp	120	0.04	0.2	0.09	0.47	0	0.05	0.46	0.3906	0.6042
	Hal	119	0.05	0.26	0.13	0.55	0	0.08	0.51	0.0859	
Dyskinesia	Arp	120	0.14	0.54	0.09	0.34	0	-0.05	0.25	0.0625	0.4114
	Hal	119	0.08	0.4	0.09	0.41	0	0.01	0.4	1	
Overall Severity	Arp	120	0.79	0.89	0.84	0.86	0	0.05	0.79	0.4592	0.0094
	Hal	119	0.71	0.82	1.03	0.99	0	0.32	0.92	0.0001	

Abbreviations: N = total number of patients with a baseline and at least one postbaseline score, SD = standard deviation, Arp = aripiprazole, Hal = haloperidol. 1. Within treatment group changes were tested with Wilcoxon signed-rank test. 2. Treatment group comparisons of change score distributions were tested with the Wilcoxon rank-sum test.

6.1.5. Comparison of EPS profiles between blonanserin and haloperidol

Inada et al. (2008) reported that blonanserin, a serotonin-dopamine antagonist developed as an atypical antipsychotic and currently available in Japan, had a more favorable EPS profile than haloperidol in a double-blind comparative study conducted in Japan. The purpose of the study was to demonstrate the superiority of blonanserin with regard to the incidence of EPS using the DIEPSS in Japanese patients with schizophrenia. A particular focus was the ability of the DIEPSS to capture differences in the EPS profiles between blonanserin, an atypical antipsychotic, and haloperidol, a conventional one.

Schizophrenic patients who met the criteria for category F20 of the ICD-10 were enrolled in this study and received 8 weeks of treatment with blonanserin or haloperidol. The dose ranges were 8-24 mg/day in the blonanserin group and 4-12 mg/day in the haloperidol group. When anticholinergics were used at study entry, these drugs were to be tapered off and terminated within 1 to 2 weeks from the baseline assessment. Preventive treatment with anticholinergics was not to be performed. The rates of concomitant use of anticholinergics and the biperiden equivalent doses were also compared between the two groups. The incidence of EPS was significantly lower in the blonanserin group than in the haloperidol group. The change in the DIEPSS total score worsened to a significantly greater extent in the haloperidol group than in the blonanserin group. Significant differences between the two groups were observed from the first week to the 6th week for the DIEPSS total scores (**Figure 5**), and from the 3rd week to the 8th week for the rate of concomitant use of anticholinergics and for the the biperiden equivalent doses (**Figure 6**). These results indicate that the favorable EPS profile of blonanserin was detectable using DIEPSS assessments from the early stage of the study.

Section 6. Clinical application of the DIEPSS

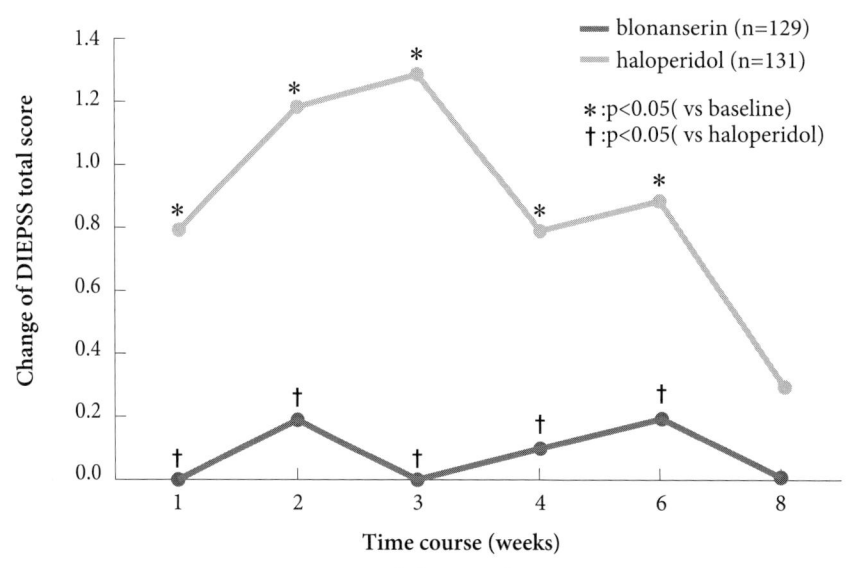

Figure 5. Time course of change of DIEPSS total score

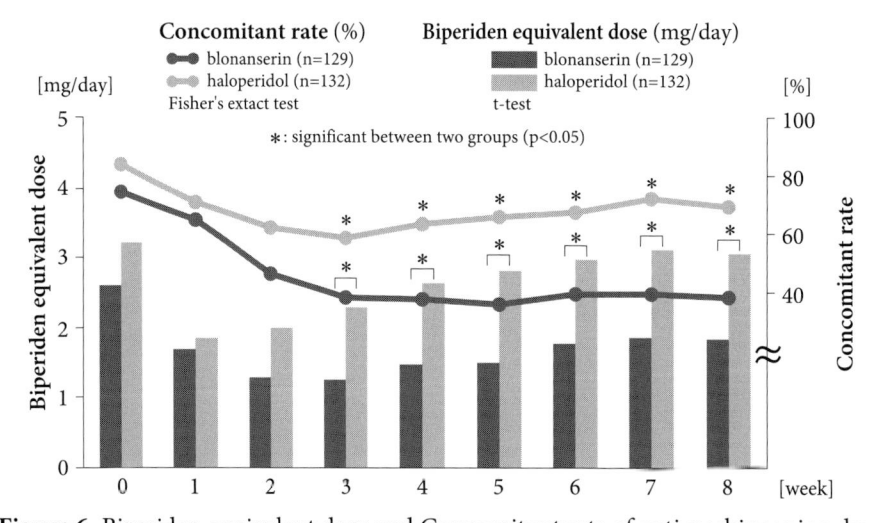

Figure 6. Biperiden equivalent dose and Concomitant rate of anti-parkinsonian drug

6.2. Preventive Strategies for EPS using the DIEPSS

Although acute or subacute EPS can be treated by reducing the dose of the antipsychotic drug or by adding an anticholinergic drug, the presence of these symptoms has been reported to increase the risk of developing irreversible or treatment-refractory TD. To avoid the appearance of severe or distressing forms of acute EPS and to prevent the later development of TD, it is essential to recognize even subtle forms of acute EPS or dyskinetic signs in the very early stages of antipsychotic treatment and to take appropriate intervention steps. If the first signs of EPS are detected during the early stages of antipsychotic treatment, it is strongly recommended that the dose of the antipsychotic drug should be decreased to the minimum effective dose. Systematic routine monitoring with an appropriate rating scale is important, and is the first step of the recommended strategy for detecting early signs of EPS and preventing their development into more serious conditions. Due to its brevity and simplicity, the DIEPSS is an ideal tool for routine screening in clinical practice, and has been recommended for detecting the early signs of EPS in schizophrenic patients from the initial phase of antipsychotic administration onward.

When EPS are observed in psychiatric patients, the first step is to identify the causative drug. Although antipsychotics are the most likely cause of EPS in schizophrenic patients, other medicines can produce these symptoms. Therefore, it is important to conduct a thorough review of all the patient's medications. Extrapyramidal symptoms can be induced or worsened by several drug groups, including benzamide substitutes such as tiapride and sulpiride, antihypertensive drugs, calcium channel blockers, histamine H2 blockers such as cimetidine, ranitidine and famotidine, antidepressants and thyroid medications. However, although EPS may develop with the use of histamine H2 blockers, the prevalence is low. Since histamine H2 blockers rarely affect dopaminergic systems, a dopamine-acetylcholine imbalance due to the inhibition of acetylcholine release has been proposed to explain the etiology. The prevalence of EPS induced by antidepressants is also low; it has been estimated at approximately 2%. Concurrent medical problems also need to be considered; for example, fever, thyroid disease, liver disease and anxiety disorder may cause or exacerbate tremor (Hubble, 2000).

Monitoring for EPS using the DIEPSS is especially important in elderly psychiatric patients receiving antipsychotic drugs because the risks of EPS increase with aging. However, the evaluation of gait and bradykinesia is sometimes difficult in elderly patients with senile motor disturbance, and virtually impossible in bed-ridden patients. The evaluation of subjective symptoms of akathisia is also difficult in elderly schizophrenic patients with impaired cognitive function. In addition, it is also difficult to differentiate antipsychotic-induced EPS from those of non-antipsychotic origin in elderly patients who showed neurological signs before the initiation of antipsychotic therapy (Inada et al, 1997).

6.3. Other clinical and biological studies

The DIEPSS has also been used for the evaluation of EPS in patients receiving antipsychotic agents in various clinical, psychopharmacological, and biological studies. Murashita et al (2007) reported low frequencies of occurrence of EPS in schizophrenic patients receiving long-term risperidone monotherapy. Matsuzawa et al (2008) examined correlations between glutathione levels and clinical variables in schizophrenic patients, and found a significant negative correlation between glutathione levels and the severity of negative symptoms. They reported that there were no significant correlations between glutathione levels and DIEPSS score. Some of the other clinical and biological studies that have used the DIEPSS are summarized in this chapter.

6.3.1. Quetiapine treatment for behavioral and psychological symptoms of dementia (BPSD) in patients with senile dementia of the Alzheimer type (SDAT)

Fujikawa et al. (2004) examined the therapeutic effects of quetiapine in the treatment of BPSD in patients with SDAT. Sixteen SDAT patients with BPSD were recruited and quetiapine (25-200 mg/day) was prescribed for 8 weeks. BPSD were evaluated using the Behavioral Pathology in Alzheimer's Disease Rating Scale (BehaveAD) and the Cohen-Mansfield Agitation Inventory (CMAI) at week 0 (baseline) and week 8 (endpoint). The severity of EPS was also assessed using the DIEPSS at baseline and at endpoint. Significant improvements were observed in the CMAI total score and in the BehaveAD subscales for delusions, activity disturbances, aggressiveness and diurnal rhythm disturbances, and in the BehaveAD overall severity score. No significant difference in the DIEPSS score was observed between the baseline and endpoint. These data indicate that quetiapine is effective in controlling BPSD and has a favorable EPS profile.

6.3.2. Correlation between reduction of EPS and improvement in quality of life (QOL)

In the validation study of the Japanese version of the Schizophrenia Quality of Life Scale (SQLS) as an assessment tool, Kaneda et al, (2002) evaluated the SQLS by comparing it with two other self-reporting measures, the Medical Outcomes Study 36-item Short-Form Health Survey questionnaire (SF-36) and the WHO QOL-26, in 55 schizophrenic inpatients. In this study, psychotic symptoms and extrapyramidal symptoms were assessed using the Brief Psychiatric Rating Scale (BPRS) and the DIEPSS, respectively. All QOL scales (psychosocial, motivation/energy and symptoms/side effects) showed good internal consistency in the reliability tests (Cronbach's alpha coefficients were 0.93, 0.73 and 0.80, respectively). The correlations of items with their scales revealed that almost all items correlated significantly with the scores within their own scale. SQLS scores also correlated well with the relevant SF-36, WHO QOL-26 and DIEPSS scores. Subsequently, Taniguchi et al. (2006) examined the correlation between the severity of EPS and QOL in a study in which the patients' existing antipsychotic drugs were replaced with quetiapine in a naturalistic setting. This was carried out in 21 chronic schizophrenic patients who still showed moderate psychiatric symptoms and either showed EPS or took anti-parkinsonian drugs for the EPS. Quetiapine was added on and gradually increased while the previous drugs were tapered and discontinued whenever possible. Clinical symptoms, objective and subjective QOL, and EPS were measured before and 6 months after quetiapine addition, using the BPRS, Quality of Life Scale (QLS), SQLS and DIEPSS, respectively. Replacement with quetiapine improved both clinical symptoms and EPS, along with objective and subjective QOL. These results suggest that the severity of EPS, as assessed by the DIEPSS, is correlated with the quality of life in schizophrenic patients receiving antipsychotic agents.

Adherence to antipsychotic treatment is particularly important in the long-term management of schizophrenia since poor adherence to medication is associated with poor health outcomes. Fujikawa et al (2008) investigated subjective satisfaction with antipsychotics in patients with schizophrenia and they reported that satisfaction with regard to side-effects and global satisfaction were significantly higher in patients taking second-generation antipsychotics than those taking first-generation antipsychotics, whereas no significant difference was found between the two groups in clinical symptoms according to BPRS or the DIEPSS.

6.3.3. Association between antipsychotic-induced EPS and polymorphisms in the dopamine D2-receptor (DRD2) gene

Nakazono et al. (2005) examined the relationship between polymorphisms in the DRD2 gene

(Taq1A, Taq1B, -141C Ins/Del) and the risk of EPS (assessed with the DIEPSS) or the maintenance dose of antipsychotics in schizophrenic patients. The DIEPSS score was significantly higher in patients bearing the -141C Del allele than in those without it. Taq1A and Taq1B restriction fragment length polymorphisms (RFLPs) did not significantly affect the DIEPSS score. On the other hand, maintenance doses of neuroleptics and antiparkinsonian drugs were significantly higher in patients with the B1 allele of the Taq1B RFLP than in those without it, while Taq1A RFLP and -141C Ins/Del polymorphisms were not significantly related to the maintenance doses. The authors concluded that the risk of EPS may be increased in patients with the -141C Del allele of the DRD2 gene. In these patients, antipsychotics should be administered with caution.

6.3.4. Serum testosterone levels and the severity of negative symptoms

It has been suggested that gonadal sex hormones play a role in the pathophysiology of schizophrenia, based on the results of recent neuroendocrinological studies. Ko et al. (2007) examined the relationship between negative symptoms and plasma levels of free testosterone, total testosterone, dehydroepiandrosterone sulfate, estradiol and prolactin, with regard to depressive symptoms, EPS and other factors including differences in age, diurnal variation of the serum hormone levels, and body fat composition in 35 male inpatients with chronic schizophrenia aged 20-39 years. The psychotic symptoms were assessed using the PANSS. The Calgary Depression Scale for Schizophrenia (CDSS) and the DIEPSS were also used to exclude the effects of depression or drug-induced movement disorders. The PANSS negative scores had a significant inverse correlation with the serum total and free testosterone levels. Moreover, a partial correlation analysis showed an inverse correlation between the PANSS negative subscores and the serum total and free testosterone levels after controlling for the DIEPSS and CDSS scores and age. These results suggest that total and free testosterone may play an important role in determining the severity of negative symptoms in male patients with schizophrenia.

References

Adler CH. Differential diagnosis of Parkinson's disease. Med Clin North Am 83: 349–367, 1999.

American Psychiatric Association. Practice guideline for the treatment of patients with schizophrenia. Am J Psychiatry 154S: 1-63, 1997.

Ayd FJ Jr. A survey of drug-induced extrapyramidal reactions. J Am Med Assoc 175: 1054-1060, 1961.

Ayd FJ Jr. Early onset neuroleptic-induced extra-pyramidal reactions: a second survey, 1961-1981. In: Coyle JT, Enna SJ, eds. Neuroleptics: Neurochemical, Behavioral, and Clinical Perspectives. New York, Raven Press, 1983.

Barnes TRE. A rating scale for drug-induced akathisia. Br J Psychiatry 154: 672-676, 1989.

Barnes TRE, Braude WM. Persistent akathisia associated with early tardive dyskinesia. Postgrad Med J 60: 51-53, 1984.

Barnes TR, Kane JM. The assessment of movement disorder in psychosis. In: Barnes TR, Nelson HE, editors. The assessment of psychoses. Chapman and Hall Medical, London: pp191–210, 1994.

Braude WM, Barnes TRE, Gore SM. Clinical characteristics of akathisia: a systematic investigation of acute psychiatric inpatient admissions. Br J Psychiatry 143: 139-150, 1983.

Burke RE, Fahn S, Jankovic J, Marsden CD, Lang AE, Gollomp S, Ilson J. Tardive dystonia: late-onset and persistent dystonia caused by antipsychotic drugs. Neurology 32: 1335–1346, 1982.

Cassady SL, Thaker GK, Summerfelt A, Tamminga CA. The Maryland Psychiatric Research Center scale and the characterization of involuntary movements. Psychiatry Res 70: 21–37, 1997.

Chouinard G, Annable L, Ross-Chouinard A, Nestoros JN. Factors related to tardive dyskinesia. Am J Psychiatry 136: 79-83, 1979.

Chouinard G, Margolese HC. Manual for the Extrapyramidal Symptom Rating Scale (ESRS). Schizophr Res 76: 247-265, 2005.

Chouinard G, Ross-Chouinard A, Annable L, Jones BD. Extrapyramidal symptom rating scale. Can J Neurol Sci 7: 233, 1980.

Conley RR. Evaluating clinical trial data: outcome measures. J Clin Psychiatry 62 (Suppl. 9): 23–26, 2001.

Fujikawa M, Togo T, Yoshimi A, Fujita J, Nomoto M, Kamijo A, Amagai T, Uchikado H, Katsuse O, Hosojima H, Sakura Y, Furusho R, Suda A, Yamaguchi T, Hori T, Kamada A, Kondo T, Ito M, Odawara T, Hirayasu Y. Evaluation of subjective treatment satisfaction with antipsychotics in schizophrenia patients. Prog Neuropsychopharmacol Biol Psychiatry 32: 755-760, 2008.

Fujikawa T, Takahashi T, Kinoshita A, Kajiyama H, Kurata A, Yamashita H, Yamawaki S. Quetiapine treatment for behavioral and psychological symptoms in patients with senile dementia of Alzheimer type. Neuropsychobiology 49: 201-204, 2004.

Gerlach J, Casey DE. Tardive dyskinesia. Acta Psychiatr Scand 77: 369-378, 1988.

Gerlach J, Korsgaard S, Clemmesen P, Lauersen AML, Magelund G, Noring U, Povlsen UJ, Bech P, Casey DE. The St. Hans Rating Scale for extrapyramidal syndromes: reliability and validity. Acta Psychiatr Scand 87: 244-252, 1993.

Giraudeau B, Mary JY. Planning a reproducibility study: how many subjects and how many replicates per subject for an expected width of the 95% confidence interval of the intraclass correlation coefficient. Stat Med 20: 3205–3214, 2001.

Guy W. ECDEU assessment manual for psychopharmacology. Bethesda, MD: U.S. Department of Health, Education, and Welfare; 1976.

Hair JF Jr, Anderson RE, Tatham RL, Black WC. Multivariate data analysis, 5th ed. New Jersey: Prentice-Hall International; 1998.

Hubble JP. Essential tremor: diagnosis and treatment. In: Adler CH, Ahlskog JE, eds. Parkinson's

Disease and Movement Disorders: Diagnosis and Treatment Guidelines for the Practicing Physician. Totowa, NJ: Humana Press, pp283–295, 2000.

Hyde TM, Egan MF, Brown RJ, Weinberger DR, Kleinman JE. Diurnal variation in tardive dyskinesia. Psychiatry Res 56: 53-57, 1995.

Inada T. Evaluation and diagnosis of drug-induced extrapyramidal symptoms: commentary on the DIEPSS and guide to its usage. Tokyo: Seiwa Shoten Publishers; 1996.

Inada T. EPS Profiles of atypical antipsychotics assessed by DIEPSS. In: (Satellite symposium) "EPS advantage" and relevant clinical benefits beyoud EPS. 12th meeting of the World Congress of Psychiatry, Yokohama, August, 2002.

Inada T, Matsuda G, Kitao Y, Nakamura A, Miyata R, Inagaki A, Koshiishi M, Kanba S and Yagi G. Barnes Akathisia Scale: usefulness of standardized videotape method in evaluation of the reliability and in training raters. Int J Meth Psychiatr Res 6: 49-52, 1996.

Inada T, Ohnishi K, Kamisada M, Matsuda G, Tajima O, Yanagisawa Y, Hashiguchi K, Shima S, Oh-e Y, Masuda Y, Chiba T, Kamijima K, Rockhold RW, Yagi G. A prospective study of tardive dyskinesia in Japan. Euro Arch Psychiatry Clin Neurosci 240: 250-254, 1991.

Inada T, Yagi G. Current topics in tardive dyskinesia in Japan. Psychiatr Clin Neurosci 49: 239–244, 1995.

Inada T, Yagi G. Current topics in neuroleptic-induced extrapyramidal symptoms in Japan. Keio J Med 45: 95-99, 1996.

Inada T, Yagi G, Miura S. Extrapyramidal symptom profiles in Japanese patients with schizophrenia treated with olanzapine or haloperidol. Schizophr Res 57: 227-38, 2002.

Inada T, Beasley CM Jr, Tanaka Y, Walker DJ. Extrapyramidal symptom profiles assessed with the Drug-induced Extrapyramidal Symptom Scale: comparison with Western scales in the clinical double-blind studies of schizophrenic patients treated with either olanzapine or haloperidol. Int Clin Psychopharmacol 18: 39-48, 2003.

Inada T, Ishigooka J, Murasaki M: Favorable extrapyramidal symptoms profile of Blonanserin, a serotonin-dopamine antagonist developed in Japan, as assessed by DIEPSS. Abstract of the 26th Collegium Internationale Neuropsychopharmacologicum (CINP), Munich, Germany, July 13-17, 2008.

Ishigooka J, Inada T, Miura S. Olanzapine versus haloperidol in the treatment of patients with chronic schizophrenia: results of the Japan multicenter, double-blind olanzapine trial. Psychiatr Clin Neurosci 55: 403-414, 2001.

Kane JM, Carson WH, Saha AR, McQuade RD, Ingenito GG, Zimbroff DL, Ali MW. Efficacy and safety of aripiprazole and haloperidol versus placebo in patients with schizophrenia and schizoaffective disorder. J Clin Psychiatry 63(9): 763-771, 2002.

Kaneda Y, Imakura A, Fujii A, Ohmori T. Schizophrenia Quality of Life Scale: validation of the Japanese version. Psychiatry Res 113: 107-13, 2002.

Kay SR, Opler LA, Fiszbein A. Positive and negative syndrome scale. Multi-Health System Inc. Tronto, Canada, 1991

Keepers GA, ClappisonVJ, Casey DE. Initial anticholinergic prophylaxis for neuroleptic-induced extrapyramidal syndromes. Arch Gen Psychiatry 40: 113-1117, 1983.

Kim JH, Jung HY, Kang UG, Jeong SH, Ahn YM, Byun HJ, Ha KS, Kim YS. Metric characteristics of the drug-induced extrapyramidal symptoms scale (DIEPSS): a practical combined rating scale for drug-induced movement disorders. Mov Disord 17: 1354-1359, 2002a.

Kim JH, Lee BC, Park HJ, Ahn YM, Kang UG, Kim YS. Subjective emotional experience and cognitive impairment in drug-induced akathisia. Compr Psychiatry 43: 456-462, 2002b.

Ko YH, Jung SW, Joe SH, Lee CH, Jung HG, Jung IK, Kim SH, Lee MS. Association between serum testosterone levels and the severity of negative symptoms in male patients with chronic schizophrenia. Psychoneuroendocrinology 32: 385-391, 2007.

References

Loonen AJ, Doorschot CH, van Hemert DA, Oostelbos MC, Sijben AE. The Schedule for the assessment of Drug-induced Movement Disorders (SADIMoD): test–retest reliability and concurrent validity. Int J Neuropsychopharmacol 3: 285–296, 2000.

Martinez-Martin P, Gil-Nagel A, Gracia LM, Gomez JB, Martinez-Sarries J, Bermejo F. Unified Parkinson's Disease Rating Scale characteristics and structure. The Cooperative Multicentric Group. Mov Disord 9: 76–83, 1994.

Matsuzawa D, Obata T, Shirayama Y, Nonaka H, Kanazawa Y, Yoshitome E, Takanashi J, Matsuda T, Shimizu E, Ikehira H, Iyo M, Hashimoto K. Negative correlation between brain glutathione level and negative symptoms in schizophrenia: a 3T 1H-MRS study. PLoS ONE 3: e1944, 2008.

McEvoy JP, Weiden PJ, Smith TE, Carpenter D, Kahn DA, Frances A (eds). The expert consensus guideline series: Treatment of schizophrenia. J Clin Psychiatry 57 (Suppl 12B): 7-58, 1996.

Murphy JM, Berwick DM, Weinstein MC, Borus JF, Budman SH, Klerman GL. Performance of screening and diagnostic tests. Application of receiver operating characteristic analysis. Arch Gen Psychiatry 44: 550–555, 1987.

Murashita M, Inoue T, Kusumi I, Nakagawa S, Itoh K, Tanaka T, Izumi T, Hosoda H, Kangawa K, Koyama T. Glucose and lipid metabolism of long-term risperidone monotherapy in patients with schizophrenia. Psychiatry Clin Neurosci 61: 54-58, 2007.

Muscettola G, Barbato G, Pampallona S, Casiello M, Bollini P. Extrapyramidal syndromes in neuroleptic-treated patients: prevalence, risk factors, and association with tardive dyskinesia. J Clin Psychopharmacol 19: 203–208, 1999.

Nakazono Y, Abe H, Murakami H, Koyabu N, Isaka Y, Nemoto Y, Murata S, Tsutsumi Y, Ohtani H, Sawada Y. Association between neuroleptic drug-induced extrapyramidal symptoms and dopamine D2-receptor polymorphisms in Japanese schizophrenic patients. Int J Clin Pharmacol Ther 43: 163-171, 2005.

Overall JE, Gorham DR: The brief psychiatric rating scale. Psychol Rep 10: 799-812, 1962.

Owens DGC. Adverse effects of antipsychotic agents- do newer agents offer advantages? Drugs 51: 895-930, 1996.

Owens DGC. A guide to the extrapyramidal side-effects of antipsychotic drugs. Cambridge: Cambridge University Press, 1999.

[No authors listed]. Treatment of schizophrenia 1999. The expert consensus guideline series. J Clin Psychiatry 60 (Suppl 11): 3-80, 1999.

Pivac N, Kozaric-Kovacic D, Muck-Seler D. Olanzapine versus fluphenazine in an open trial in patients with psychotic combat-related post-traumatic stress disorder. Psychopharmacology (Berl) 175: 451-456, 2004.

Rabey JM, Bass H, Bonuccelli U, Brooks D, Klotz P, Korczyn AD, Kraus P, Martinez-Martin P, Morrish P, Van Sauten W, Van Hilten B. Evaluation of the Short Parkinson's Evaluation Scale: a new friendly scale for the evaluation of Parkinson's disease in clinical drug trials. Clin Neuropharmacol 20: 322–337, 1997.

Rifkin A, Quitkin F, Klein DF. Akinesia. A poorly recognized drug-induced extrapyramidal behavioral disorder. Arch Gen Psychiatry 32: 672-674, 1975.

Sachdev P, Kruk J. Clinical characteristics and predisposing factors in acute drug-induced akathisia. Arch Gen Psychiatry 51: 963–974, 1994.

Schooler NR, Kane JM. Research diagnoses for tardive dyskinesia. Arch Gen Psychiatry 39: 486–487, 1982.

Simpson GM, Angus JWS. A rating scale for extrapyramidal side effects. Acta Psychiatr Scand 45 (Suppl 212): 11-19, 1970.

Siris SG. Akinesia and Postpsychotic depression: A difficult differential diagnosis. J Clin Psychiatry 48: 240-243, 1987.

Siris SG. Three cases of akathisia and "acting-out." J Clin Psychiatry 46: 395-397, 1985.

Taniguchi T, Sumitani S, Aono M, Iga J, Kinouchi S, Aki H, Matsushita M, Taniguchi K, Tsuno M, Yamanishi K, Tomotake M, Kaneda Y, Ohmori T. Effect of antipsychotic replacement with quetiapine on the symptoms and quality of life of schizophrenic patients with extrapyramidal symptoms. Hum Psychopharmacol 21: 439-445, 2006.

Tarsy D. Neuroleptic-induced extrapyramidal reactions: classification, description, and diagnosis. Clin Neuropharmacol 6 (Suppl 1), 9-26, 1983.

Tarsy D. Akathisia. In: Joseph AB, Young RR eds. Movement disorders in neurology and neuropsychiatry. Blackwell Scientific Publications, Boston: pp88-99, 1992.

van Harten PN, Hoek HW, Matroos GE, Koeter M, Kahn RS. The inter-relationships of tardive dyskinesia, Parkinsonism, akathisia, and tardive dystonia: the Curacao Extrapyramidal Syndromes Study II. Schizophr Res 26: 235–242, 1997.

van Harten PN, Kahn RS. Tardive dystonia. Schizophr Bull 25: 741-748, 1999.

van Putten T. The many faces of akathisia. Compr Psychiatry 16: 43-47, 1975.

van Putten T, May PRA. 'Akinetic depression' in schizophrenia. Arch Gen Psychiatry 35: 1101-1107, 1978.

Appendix

Ⅰ. Japanese version

Ⅱ. Chinese version

Ⅲ. Taiwanese version

Ⅳ. Korean version

Ⅴ. English version

Appendix I - Japanese version

DIEPSS（薬原性錐体外路症状評価尺度）評価者用マニュアル

　この評価尺度表は抗精神病薬の治療中に発症する薬原性錐体外路症状の重症度を評価するために作成されたものであり，8つの個別評価項目と1つの総括評価項目からなりたっている。評価者は医学のトレーニングを積んでおり，神経学的症状評価についての十分な知識も持っていることが必要であり，かつ安定したデータが得られるようになるために本評価尺度表を使用するにあたっての十分な訓練を受けた者でなければならない。評価者は原則として被験者を直接診察することによって，診察中に観察される症状から被験者の評価にあたるが，病棟スタッフや家族からの情報も考慮にいれる。振戦，アカシジア，ジストニアなどの個別項目では，評価時に観察されない症状が夕薬服用後や就寝前のみに出現するといった，評価時以外の特定の時間帯に限局して出現すると訴える場合もあり，このような症例では被験者との問診や病棟スタッフや家族から得られる情報を考慮に入れて，その症状の重症度について注意深く評価すべきである。各研究プロトコールで定められた期間内（たとえば最近24時間以内，3日以内など）に観察される最も重篤な症状がその評価対象となる。以下の用語解説は特定の項目を評価するためのガイドラインを示したものである。

1 ｜ 歩行　Gait

　被験者に普段その被験者が道を歩くときと同じように歩いてもらう。ここでは，歩行の遅さ，すなわち速度の低下，歩幅の減少，上肢の振れの減少の程度についての評価を行い，前屈姿勢，前方突進現象の程度も考慮すること。これらの重症度が一致しない場合には，観察された症状の中から，最も重篤な症状に重点を置いて評価すること。また，歩行の開始困難や終了困難の程度は動作緩慢の項目を評価する際にも考慮すること。

- 0＝正常。
- 1＝上肢の振りがわずかに少なく，速度や歩幅もわずかに減少した歩行という印象。
- 2＝歩行速度や歩幅の軽度減少，および上肢の振りの軽度低下。軽度の前屈姿勢が観察される場合もある。
- 3＝上肢の振りがかなり減少した明らかに遅い歩行。典型的な前屈姿勢と小刻みな歩行。時に前方突進現象が認められる。
- 4＝一人での歩行開始はほとんど不可能。いったん歩行が開始されても非常に小刻みな歩行で引きずるように歩き，上肢の振りは全く見られない。重度の前方突進現象のみられることがある。

2 ｜ 動作緩慢　Bradykinesia

　動作が鈍くなったり，遅くなったりして，活動性が乏しくなること。動作の開始が遅延し，時には困難になる。顔面の表情の変化の乏しさの程度（仮面様顔貌），評価面接の際の話し方（単調で緩徐な話し方）についても評価すること。

- 0＝正常。
- 1＝動作が緩慢であるという印象。
- 2＝軽度の動作緩慢。わずかに認められる動作の開始または終了の遅延。会話のテンポはやや緩徐で，顔面の表情も幾分乏しい。
- 3＝中等度の動作緩慢。動作の開始または終了に明らかな困難をきたす。会話のテンポは中等度に遅く，顔面の表情変化も中等度に乏しい。
- 4＝重度の動作緩慢，もしくは不動（アキネジア）。被験者はほとんど動かない，または移動の際に多大な努力を要する。顔面表情筋の動きはほとんど見られず（典型的な仮面様顔貌），会話のテンポも著しく遅い。

3 ｜ 流涎　Sialorrhea

唾液分泌過多の程度を評価すること。

- 0＝正常。
- 1＝評価面接の際にみられるごく軽度の唾液分泌過多の印象。
- 2＝評価面接の際にみられる口内にたまる軽度の唾液分泌過多。ほとんど会話の障害にはならない。
- 3＝評価面接の際にみられる中等度の唾液分泌過多。このためしばしば会話に困難を伴う。
- 4＝絶えず認められる重度の流涎，または垂れ流しの状態。

4 ｜ 筋強剛　Muscle rigidity

上肢の屈伸に対する抵抗の程度を評価する。歯車現象，ろう屈現象や手首の曲がり具合の程度も評価すること。

0＝なし。
1＝上肢の屈伸でごく軽度の抵抗を感じるという印象。
2＝上肢の屈伸における軽度の抵抗。軽度の歯車現象が時に認められる。
3＝上肢の屈伸における中等度の抵抗。明らかな歯車現象のみられることがある。
4＝上肢の屈伸に非常に強い力を要し，中断するとそのままの肢位を保つ（ろう屈現象）。重度の筋強剛のためにしばしば上肢の屈伸が困難となることもある。

5 ｜ 振戦　Tremor

口部，手指，四肢，躯幹に認められる反復的，規則的で（４～８Ｈｚ），リズミカルな運動。客観的に観察される症状の出現頻度やその重症度に重点を置いて評価するが，そのために被験者の感じる苦痛や日常生活への影響の程度も考慮すること。

0＝なし。
1＝非特異的で軽微な振戦。または断続的に認められる一部位に限局した軽度の振戦。
2＝一部位に限局した軽度の振戦が持続的に観察される。または複数の部位にまたがる軽度の振戦，あるいは一部位に限局した中等度の振戦が断続的に認められる。
3＝一部位に限局した中等度の振戦が持続的に観察される。または複数の部位にまたがる中等度の振戦，あるいは一部位に限局した重度の振戦が断続的に認められる。
4＝重度の全般性振戦，または全身の粗大振戦

6 ｜ アカシジア　Akathisia

アカシジアは静座不能に対する自覚，下肢のムズムズ感，ソワソワ感，絶えず動いていたいという衝動などの自覚的な内的不穏症状と，それに付随してみられる身体の揺り動かし，下肢の振り回し，足踏み，足の組み換え，ウロウロ歩きなどの客観的な運動亢進症状から成る。その評価にあたっては自覚症状の程度を優先して評価し，運動亢進症状は，主観症状を支持する所見として用いること。たとえば，アカシジアに特徴的な運動不穏の症状が顕著に認められても，内的不穏の自覚がない場合には０，非特異的ではっきりしない場合には１と評価する（仮性アカシジア）。アカシジアの評価に際しては，評価面接全体を通しての落ち着きのなさの有無も考慮に入れること。

0＝なし
1＝非特異的で軽微な内的不穏感。
2＝内的不穏に対する軽度の自覚はあるが，それは必ずしも苦痛の原因にはなっていない。アカシジアに特徴的な運動亢進症状の観察されることがある。
3＝中等度の内的不穏。このため不快な症状や苦痛が認められる。主観的な内的不穏に基づく身体の揺り動かし，下肢の振り回し，足踏みなどの下肢の特徴的な運動不穏が観察される。
4＝重度の内的不穏があり，このため被験者はじっとしていることができず，絶えず下肢を動かしている。睡眠障害や不安感を伴うことがある明らかに苦痛な状態。被験者はそれらの症状の鎮静を強く望む。

7 │ ジストニア　Dystonia

ジストニアは舌，頚部，四肢，躯幹などにみられる突発的な筋肉の捻転やつっぱり，痙縮あるいは持続的な異常ポジションで示されるような，筋緊張の異常な亢進によって引き起こされる症状の一群である。この症状に含まれるものには，舌の突出捻転，斜頚，後頚，牙関緊急，眼球上転，ピサ症候群などがある。ここでは筋緊張の亢進異常の程度を評価の対象とし，ジストニアで誘発される異常運動の程度はジスキネジアの項目で評価すること。客観的に観察される症状の出現頻度やその重症度に重点を置いて評価するが，ジストニアのために被験者の感じる苦痛や日常生活への影響の程度も考慮すること。嚥下困難や舌の肥厚などの付随する症状もこの項目を評価する際に考慮すること。

- 0＝なし。
- 1＝軽微な筋肉のこわばり，捻転，異常ポジションがあるという印象。
- 2＝軽度のジストニア。舌，頚部，四肢，躯幹にみられる軽度の捻転やつっぱり，痙縮，または軽度の眼球上転。被験者は必ずしも苦痛を感じていない。
- 3＝中等度のジストニア。中等度の捻転やつっぱり，痙縮，眼球上転。被験者はしばしばその症状に対する苦痛を訴える。迅速な治療が望まれる。
- 4＝四肢や躯幹に認められる重度のジストニア。このため食事や歩行などの日常生活の活動に著しい支障をきたす。可及的すみやかな治療の適応となる。

8 │ ジスキネジア　Dyskinesia

運動の異常に亢進した状態。顔面（顔面の表情筋），口部（口唇と口周辺部），舌，顎，上肢（腕，手首，手，指），下肢（脚，膝，踵，足趾），躯幹（頚部，肩部，臀部）にみられる他覚的に無目的で不規則な不随意運動。舞踏病様運動，アテトーゼ様運動は評価対象となるが，振戦は含まない。客観的に観察される異常不随意運動の出現頻度やその重症度に重点を置いて評価するが，異常不随意運動のために被験者の感じる苦痛や日常生活への影響の程度も考慮すること。誘発により発現する運動は自然に観察される運動よりも1ランク下げて評価すること。

- 0＝なし。
- 1＝非特異的で軽微な異常不随意運動が認められる。限局した軽度の異常不随意運動が断続的に認められる。
- 2＝限局した軽度の異常不随意運動が持続的に観察される。または複数の部位にまたがる軽度の異常不随意運動や限局した中等度以上の異常不随意運動が断続的に認められる。
- 3＝限局した中等度の異常不随意運動が持続的に観察される。または複数の部位にまたがる中等度の異常不随意運動や限局した重度の異常不随意運動が断続的に認められる。
- 4＝重度の異常不随意運動が観察される。このため日常生活に支障をきたす。

9 │ 概括重症度　Overall severity

個々の症状の重症度や出現頻度，それらの症状による苦痛の程度，日常生活への影響，さらにそれらの症状に対する処置の必要性などを考慮に入れて，錐体外路症状全体の概括重症度を評価すること。

- 0＝なし。
- 1＝ごく軽度。または疑わしい。
- 2＝軽度。日常生活にほとんど影響なし。必ずしも苦痛を感じない。
- 3＝中等度。日常生活にある程度の影響を及ぼす。しばしば苦痛を感じる。
- 4＝重度。日常生活に重大な影響を及ぼす。強く苦痛を感じる。

© Toshiya INADA, M.D.

Appendix I - Japanese version

DIEPSS（薬原性錐体外路症状評価尺度）全項目評価用紙

研究：	コード：
患者：	0 ＝ なし，正常　None, Normal
評価者：	1 ＝ ごく軽度，不確実　Minimal, Questionable
評価日：　　　年　　月　　日	2 ＝ 軽度　Mild
評価時間：　　　〜	3 ＝ 中等度　Moderate
アンカーポイントの詳細な説明については，DIEPSS の評価者用マニュアルを熟読すること。	4 ＝ 重度　Severe

適当なもの1つに〇をつける。

1　歩行　Gait
小刻みな遅い歩き方。速度の低下，歩幅の減少，上肢の振れの減少，前屈姿勢や前方突進現象の程度を評価する。

Shuffling, slow gait. Evaluate the degree of reduction in speed and step, decrease in pendular arm movement, stooped posture and propulsion phenomenon.

0　1　2　3　4

2　動作緩慢　Bradykinesia
動作がのろく乏しいこと。動作の開始または終了の遅延または困難。顔面の表情変化の乏しさ（仮面様顔貌）や単調で緩徐な話し方の程度も評価する。

Slowness and poverty of movements: Delay and/or difficulty in initiating and/or terminating movements. Rate degree of poverty of facial expression (mask-like face) and monotonous, slurred speech, as well.

0　1　2　3　4

3　流涎　Sialorrhea
唾液分泌過多。

Excess salivation.

0　1　2　3　4

4　筋強剛　Muscle rigidity
上肢の屈伸に対する抵抗。歯車現象，ろう屈現象，鉛管様強剛や手首の曲がり具合の程度も評価する。

Resistance to flexion and extension of upper arms. Rate cogwheeling, waxy flexibility, lead-pipe rigidity and the degree of flexibility of wrists, as well.

0　1　2　3　4

5　振戦　Tremor
口部，手指，四肢，躯幹に認められる反復的，規則的(4〜8 Hz)で，リズミカルな運動。

Repetitive, regular (4-8 Hz), and rhythmic movements observed in the oral region, fingers, extremities, and trunk.

0　1　2　3　4

6　アカシジア　Akathisia
静座不能に対する自覚；下肢のムズムズ感，ソワソワ感，絶えず動いていたいという衝動などの内的不穏症状とそれに関連した苦痛。運動亢進症状（身体の揺り動かし，下肢の振り回し，足踏み，足の組み換え，ウロウロ歩きなど）についても評価する。

Subjective inner restlessness and related distress; awareness of the inability to remain seated, restless legs, fidgety feelings, desire to move constantly, etc. Rate increased motor phenomena (body rocking, shifting from foot to foot, stamping in place, crossing and uncrossing legs, pacing around, etc.), as well.

0　1　2　3　4

7　ジストニア　Dystonia
筋緊張の異常な亢進によって引き起こされる症状。舌，頚部，四肢，躯幹などにみられる筋肉の捻転やつっぱり，持続的な異常ポジション。舌の突出捻転，斜頚，後頚，牙関緊急，眼球上転，ピサ症候群などを評価する。

Symptoms induced by the hypertonic state of muscles. Stiffness, twisting, and persistent abnormal position of muscles observed in tongue, neck, extremities, trunk, etc. Rate tongue protrusion, torticollis, retrocollis, trismus, oculogyric crisis, Pisa syndrome, etc.

0　1　2　3　4

8　ジスキネジア　Dyskinesia
運動の異常に亢進した状態。顔面，口部，舌，顎，四肢，躯幹にみられる他覚的に無目的で不規則な不随意運動。舞踏病様運動，アテトーゼ様運動は含むが，振戦は評価しない。

Hyperkinetic abnormal movements. Apparently purposeless, irregular, and involuntary movements observed in face, mouth, tongue, jaw, extremities and/or trunk. Include choreic and athetoid movements, but do not rate tremor.

0　1　2　3　4

9　概括重症度　Overall severity
錐体外路症状全体の重症度。

Overall severity of extrapyramidal symptoms.

0　1　2　3　4

© Toshiya INADA, M.D.

DIEPSS（药源性锥体外系症状量表）评分手册

设计这个药源性锥体外系症状量表的目的是为了评估药物引起的锥体外系症状的严重程度，这些症状是在用抗精神病药物治疗期间发生的，这个量表包括8个单项和1项总体严重程度。评分员应接受过医学培训，有充分的知识，能够评价神经系统症状。在本量表的用法方面，评分员也要接受充分的培训，以便能够重复得出稳定可靠的数据。评分员要评价受试者的症状，这些症状主要是通过与受试者直接交谈以及在交谈过程中观察发现的。评分员还要考虑病房工作人员和受试者亲属提供的信息。评价震颤、静坐不能、肌张力障碍等单项时，受试者可能会报告只在某些时间出现症状，如在晚上吃药后或睡觉前出现，而不在评价问诊当时。在这种情况下，评分员要仔细评价症状的严重程度，评价时既要考虑与受试者谈话获取的信息，也要考虑病房工作人员和受试者亲属提供的信息。要按各研究方案规定的评定时段（如最近24小时、最近3天等）所见的最重症状进行评分。各项评分标准如下。

1 | 步态　Gait

让受试者按照平常在大街上走路的方式走动。这一项要评定步态缓慢的情况，也就是评定步行速度减缓和步幅缩短的程度，以及手臂摆动幅度减少的程度。还要评定前屈姿势和前冲表现的程度。如果这些症状的强度都与参照点不一致，就优先评定受试者最重的症状。评定运动迟缓这一项时，还要考虑开始或结束走动时的困难程度。

0 = 正常。
1 = 步行速度略微减缓，步幅略微缩短，手臂摆动幅度略微减少。
2 = 步行速度轻度减缓，步幅轻度缩短，手臂摆动幅度轻度减少。有些人还有轻度的前屈。
3 = 步行速度明显减缓，手臂摆动幅度大大减少。出现典型的前屈姿势和小碎步。有时可见前冲表现。
4 = 一个人几乎不可能开步走路。即使能够开步走路，受试者也是步态拖曳，步幅非常小，手臂也不摆动。可见重度前冲表现。

2 | 运动迟缓　Bradykinesia

由于动作缓慢和缺少运动，活动减少。动作启动比较缓慢，有时会有困难。在检查期间，还要评定面部表情缺乏（面具脸）的程度，评定言语异常（说话音单调、不清）的程度。

0 = 正常。
1 = 动作缓慢。
2 = 轻度运动迟缓。动作变慢，肌张力丧失。动作启动和/或中止略微迟缓。面部表情轻度减少，语速轻度减慢。
3 = 中度运动迟缓。动作启动和/或中止明显迟缓。语速中度减慢，面部表情中度减少。
4 = 重度运动迟缓，或不能运动。受试者很少活动，或活动非常费力。面部表情几乎没什么变化（典型的面具脸）。语速明显减慢。

3 | 流涎　Sialorrhea

评定唾液过多的程度。

0 = 正常。
1 = 检查期间唾液略多。
2 = 检查期间口中唾液轻度过多。说话稍微有点困难。
3 = 检查期间唾液中度过多。常常造成说话困难。
4 = 唾液重度过多，或流口水，连续不断。

4 | 肌肉强直　Muscle rigidity

评定对手臂屈伸运动阻抗的严重程度。还要评定齿轮样强直、蜡样屈曲以及腕关节的灵活度。

0 = 无。
1 = 手臂屈伸运动略有阻力。
2 = 手臂屈伸运动有轻度阻力。有时可见轻度齿轮样强直。
3 = 手臂屈伸运动有中度阻力。可发生比较明显的齿轮样强直。
4 = 手臂屈伸运动阻力极大。一旦被打断，受试者可保持某种姿势（蜡样屈曲）。有时由于肌肉极度强直，导致手臂不能屈伸。

5 | 震颤　Tremor

反复、有规律(4-8Hz)的节律性运动，见于口部、手指、四肢和躯干部位。评定重点是客观症状的发生频率和严重程度，但也要考虑受试者主诉的痛苦程度以及症状对受试者生活质量影响的程度。

0 = 无。
1 = 同一个部位间断有轻微的非特异性震颤，和/或轻度震颤。
2 = 同一个部位持续有轻度震颤。≥2个区域间断有轻度震颤，和/或同一个部位间断有中度震颤。
3 = 同一个部位持续有中度震颤。≥2个区域间断有中度震颤，和/或同一个部位间断有重度震颤。
4 = 重度广泛震颤，和/或全身震颤。

6 | 静坐不能　Akathisia

静坐不能既包括主观感觉心神不定，如觉得不能坐下来，腿不停地动，坐立不安，不停地想动；也包括运动增多的客观表现，如身体摇晃、两脚不停地换位、原地踏步、腿不停地翘起来又放下、四处走动。评定的重点是主观症状的严重程度，并用运动增多的表现作为证据，支持主观症状。例如，如果没有心神不定，就评为0分；如果只有非特异性、不明确的心神不定，就评为1分，即使有静坐不能的不安运动典型表现（假性静坐不能），也评为1分。评定静坐不能时，还要考虑整个检查期间有没有心神不定。

0 = 无。
1 = 轻微的非特异性心神不定。
2 = 轻度心神不定，不一定会导致主观的痛苦。可见静坐不能的运动增多典型表现。
3 = 中度心神不定。导致不适症状和痛苦。由于心神不定，出现腿不停地动典型表现，如身体摇晃、两脚不停地换位及原地踏步。
4 = 重度心神不定。导致坐不下来，或腿不停地动。非常痛苦，可妨碍睡眠，和/或引起焦虑状态。受试者非常想消除这些症状。

7 | 肌张力障碍　Dystonia

肌张力障碍是由肌张力亢进引起的综合征，表现有肌肉僵硬、扭曲、痉挛、收缩和位置持续异常，见于舌、颈部、四肢、躯干等部位。症状包括吐舌、斜颈、颈后倾、牙关紧闭、眼动危象、Pisa综合征等。这一项只评定肌张力增加的异常程度。肌张力障碍所致运动异常的程度应当按运动障碍评定。评定的重点是客观症状的发生频率和严重程度，但也要考虑受试者主诉的痛苦程度以及症状对受试者生活质量影响的程度。进行这项评定时，要考虑到伴发症状，如受试者主诉的吞咽困难、舌的厚度等。

0 = 无。
1 = 肌肉轻微发紧、扭曲或姿势异常。
2 = 轻度肌张力障碍。舌、颈部、四肢、躯干轻度僵硬、扭曲或痉挛，或有轻度眼动危象。受试者不一定会觉得痛苦。
3 = 中度肌张力障碍。肌肉中度僵硬、扭曲、收缩，或有中度眼动危象。受试者常常说这些症状使其感觉痛苦。希望迅速得到治疗。
4 = 躯干和/或四肢有重度肌张力障碍。由于有这些症状，受试者的日常活动很困难，如吃饭和走路。迫切需要立即治疗。

8 | 运动障碍　Dyskinesia

异常运动过多。运动看起来没有目的，没有规律，属于不随意运动，见于面部（面部表情肌）、口部（口唇和口周边区域）、舌、下颌、上肢（手臂、腕部、手、手指）、下肢（腿、膝部、踝部、脚趾）和/或躯干（颈部、肩部、臀部）。要评定舞蹈症样运动和手足徐动症样运动，但不包括震颤。评定的重点是客观异常不随意运动的发生频率和严重程度，但也要考虑受试者主诉的痛苦程度以及症状对受试者生活质量影响的程度。评定更多观察到的自发运动障碍，而不是需要激发后出现的运动障碍。

0 = 无。
1 = 轻微的、非特异性、异常的不随意运动。局部间断的，有轻度、异常的不随意运动。
2 = 局部持续有轻度、异常的不随意运动。≥2个区域间断有轻度、异常的不随意运动，和/或局部间断有中度、异常的不随意运动。
3 = 局部持续有中度、异常的不随意运动。≥2个区域间断有中度、异常的不随意运动轻度，和/或局部间断有重度、异常的不随意运动。
4 = 重度、异常的不随意运动。由于有这些症状，受试者的日常活动比较困难。

9 | 总体严重程度　Overall severity

评定锥体外系症状的总体严重程度，既要考虑各个症状的严重程度和发生频率，也要考虑受试者主诉的痛苦程度，考虑这些症状对受试者日常活动影响的程度，以及考虑治疗的必要性。

0 = 无。
1 = 轻微或不确定。
2 = 轻度。对受试者的日常活动几乎没有影响。不一定会感觉痛苦。
3 = 中度。对受试者的日常活动有一定程度的影响。常常会感觉痛苦。
4 = 重度。对受试者的日常活动有相当大的影响。感觉非常痛苦。

© Chinese version Qiuqing Ang, M.D./ English version Toshiya Inada, M.D.

Appendix II - Chinese version

DIEPSS（药源性锥体外系症状量表）所有项目评定用纸

研究：_____

病人：_____

评价的人：_____

评价日：_____ 年 _____ 月 _____ 日

评价时间：_____ ～ _____

关于锚点数的详细说明，请仔细阅读DIEPSS评定者用说明书。

代码：

0 ＝ 无，正常 None, Normal
1 ＝ 轻微或不确实 Minimal, Questionable
2 ＝ 轻度 Mild
3 ＝ 中度 Moderate
4 ＝ 重度 Severe

请圈出适当的一项

1 步态 Gait
步态拖曳、缓慢。评价步行速度减缓和步幅缩短的程度，评价手臂摆动减少的程度，评价前屈姿势和前冲表现的程度。
Shuffling, slow gait. Evaluate the degree of reduction in speed and step, decrease in pendular arm movement, stooped posture and propulsion phenomenon.
　　　　0　1　2　3　4

2 运动迟缓 Bradykinesia
动作缓慢，活动很少：动作开始和/或结束比较迟缓，和/或有困难。评定面部表情缺乏（面具脸）的程度，评定说话音单调、不清的程度。
Slowness and poverty of movements: Delay and/or difficulty in initiating and/or terminating movements. Rate degree of poverty of facial expression (mask-like face) and monotonous, slurred speech, as well.
　　　　0　1　2　3　4

3 流涎 Sialorrhea
唾液过多。
Excess salivation.
　　　　0　1　2　3　4

4 肌肉强直 Muscle rigidity
上臂屈伸运动有阻力。评定齿轮样强直、蜡样屈曲、铅管样强直以及腕关节的灵活度。
Resistance to flexion and extension of upper arms. Rate cogwheeling, waxy flexibility, lead-pipe rigidity and the degree of flexibility of wrists, as well.
　　　　0　1　2　3　4

5 震颤 Tremor
反复、有规律(4-8Hz)的节律性运动，见于口部、手指、四肢和躯干这些部位。
Repetitive, regular (4-8 Hz), and rhythmic movements observed in the oral region, fingers, extremities, and trunk.
　　　　0　1　2　3　4

6 静坐不能 Akathisia
主观感觉心神不定，很痛苦，觉得坐不下来，腿不停地动，坐立不安，不停地想动等表现。还要评定运动增多的表现(身体摇晃、两脚不停地换位、原地踏步、腿不停地翘起来又放下、四处走动等)。
Subjective inner restlessness and related distress; awareness of the inability to remain seated, restless legs, fidgety feelings, desire to move constantly, etc. Rate increased motor phenomena (body rocking, shifting from foot to foot, stamping in place, crossing and uncrossing legs, pacing around, etc.), as well.
　　　　0　1　2　3　4

7 肌张力障碍 Dystonia
肌张力亢进诱发的症状。肌肉僵硬、扭曲、位置持续异常，见于舌、颈部、四肢、躯干等部位。评定吐舌、斜颈、颈后倾、牙关紧闭、眼动危象、Pisa综合征等表现。
Symptoms induced by the hypertonic state of muscles. Stiffness, twisting, and persistent abnormal position of muscles observed in tongue, neck, extremities, trunk, etc. Rate tongue protrusion, torticollis, retrocollis, trismus, oculogyric crisis, Pisa syndrome, etc.
　　　　0　1　2　3　4

8 运动障碍 Dyskinesia
异常运动过多。运动看起来没有目的，没有规律，属于不随意运动，见于面部、口部、舌、下颌、四肢和/或躯干。包括舞蹈症样运动和手足徐动症样运动，但不需评价震颤。
Hyperkinetic abnormal movements. Apparently purposeless, irregular, and involuntary movements observed in face, mouth, tongue, jaw, extremities and/or trunk. Include choreic and athetoid movements, but do not rate tremor.
　　　　0　1　2　3　4

9 总体严重程度 Overall severity
锥体外系症状的总体严重程度。
Overall severity of extrapyramidal symptoms.
　　　　0　1　2　3　4

© Chinese version Qiuqing Ang, M.D./ English version Toshiya Inada, M.D.

DIEPSS（藥源性錐體外症狀量表）評分手冊

設計這個藥源性錐體外症狀量表的目的是為了評估藥物引起的錐體外症狀的嚴重程度，這些症狀是在使用抗精神病藥物治療期間發生的，這個量表包括8個單項和1項總體嚴重程度。評量員應接受過醫學培訓，有充分的知識，能夠評量神經系統症狀。在本量表的用法方面，評量員也要接受充分的培訓，以便能穩定地評量出可靠的數據。受試者的症狀評量主要以直接會談以及在會談過程中的觀察。評量員也要參考病房工作人員和受試者親屬提供的資訊。評量顫抖、靜坐不能、肌張力異常等單項時，受試者可能會報告只在某些時間出現症狀，如在晚上吃藥後或睡覺前出現，而不在評量會談當時。在這種情況下，評量員要仔細評量症狀的嚴重程度，評量時既要考慮與受試者談話獲取的信息，也要參考病房工作人員和受試者親屬提供的資訊。按照各研究方案所規定的評量時段（如最近24小時、最近3天等）所出現最重症狀評定分數。各項評分標準如下。

1 | 步態 Gait

讓受試者按照平常在馬路上走路的方式走動。這一項要評量步態緩慢的情況，也就是評量步行速度減緩和步幅縮短的程度，以及手臂擺動幅度減少的程度。還要評量前屈（駝背）姿勢和前衝現象的程度。如果這些症狀強度無法符合參照點的敘述，就優先評量受試者最重的症狀。患者出現開始或結束走動困難時，也要納入運動遲緩此項的評估。

0 = 正常。
1 = 步行速度略微減緩，步幅略微縮短，手臂擺動幅度略微減少。
2 = 步行速度輕度減緩，步幅輕度縮短，手臂擺動幅度輕度減少。有些人還有輕度的前屈。
3 = 步行速度明顯減緩，手臂擺動幅度大大減少。出現典型的前屈姿勢和小碎步。有時可見前衝表現。
4 = 幾乎無法開始走路。即使能夠開始走路，受試者也是步態拖曳，步幅非常小，手臂也不擺動。可見重度前衝表現。

2 | 運動遲緩 Bradykinesia

由於動作緩慢和缺乏，活動量減少。動作開始比較緩慢，有時會有困難。在會談過程，也要評量缺乏臉部表情（面具臉）和言語（說話音腔單調、不清）的程度。

0 = 正常。
1 = 動作緩慢的印象。
2 = 輕度運動遲緩。動作變慢，肌張力喪失。動作開始和/或結束略微遲緩。面部表情輕度減少，語速輕度減慢。
3 = 中度運動遲緩。動作開始和/或結束明顯障礙。語速中度減慢，面部表情中度減少。
4 = 重度運動遲緩，或不能運動。受試者很少活動，或活動非常費力。面部表情幾乎沒什麼變化（典型的面具臉）。語速明顯減慢。

3 | 流涎 Sialorrhea

評量唾液過多的程度。

0 = 正常。
1 = 會談期間唾液略多。
2 = 會談期間口中唾液輕度過多。說話稍微有點困難。
3 = 會談期間唾液中度過多。常常造成說話困難。
4 = 唾液重度過多，或流口水，連續不斷。

4 | 肌肉僵硬　Muscle rigidity

評量對手臂屈伸運動阻抗的嚴重程度。還要評量齒輪樣僵直、蠟樣屈曲以及腕關節的靈活度。

0 = 無。
1 = 手臂屈伸運動略有阻力。
2 = 手臂屈伸運動有輕度阻力。有時可見輕度齒輪樣僵直。
3 = 手臂屈伸運動有中度阻力。可發生比較明顯的齒輪樣僵直。
4 = 手臂屈伸運動阻力極大。一旦被打斷，受試者可保持某種姿勢（蠟樣屈曲）。有時由於肌肉極度僵直，導致手臂不能屈伸。

5 | 顫抖　Tremor

反覆、規則(4-8Hz)和具節律性的運動，見於口部、手指、四肢和軀幹部位。評量重點是客觀症狀的發生頻率和嚴重程度，但也要考慮受試者主訴的痛苦程度以及症狀對受試者生活品質影響的程度。

0 = 無。
1 = 非特異性的極輕微顫抖，和/或同一個部位間歇性觀察到輕度顫抖。
2 = 同一個部位觀察到持續輕度顫抖。兩個或以上部位出現輕度顫抖，和/或單一個部位出現間斷中度顫抖。
3 = 同一個部位觀察到持續中度顫抖。兩個或以上部位出現中度顫抖，和/或單一個部位出現間斷重度顫抖。
4 = 重度廣泛性顫抖，和/或全身震顫。

6 | 靜坐不能　Akathisia

靜坐不能既包含主觀感受到坐立不安，如覺得不能坐住，腿不停地動，忐忑不安的感覺，不停地想動；也包括運動增多的客觀表現，如身體搖晃、兩腳不停地換位、原地踏步、腿不停地翹起來又放下、四處走動。評量的重點是主觀症狀的嚴重程度，並用運動增多的表現作為證據，支持主觀症狀。例如，如果沒有坐立不安，就評為0分；如果只有非特異性、不明確的坐立不安，就評為1分，即使有靜坐不能的不安運動典型表現（假性靜坐不能）。評量靜坐不能時，還要考慮整個檢查期間有沒有坐立不安。

0 = 無。
1 = 輕微的非特異性坐立不安。
2 = 輕度坐立不安，不一定會導致主觀的痛苦。可見靜坐不能的運動增多典型表現。
3 = 中度坐立不安。導致不適症狀和痛苦。由於坐立不安，出現雙腿不停運動的典型表現，如身體搖晃、兩腳不停地換位及原地踏步。
4 = 重度坐立不安。導致無法靜坐，或雙腿不停地動。在嚴重痛苦狀況，可能會妨礙睡眠，和/或引起焦慮狀態。受試者非常想消除這些症狀。

7 | 肌張力異常　Dystonia

　　肌張力障礙是由肌張力亢進引起的症候群，表現有肌肉群的僵硬、扭曲、痙攣、收縮和持續方位異常，見於舌、頸部、四肢、軀幹等部位。症狀包括吐舌、斜頸、頸後傾、牙關緊閉、眼球上吊、比薩症候群等。這一項只評量肌張力異常增加的程度。肌張力障礙所致運動異常的程度應當按運動障礙評量。評量的重點是客觀症狀的發生頻率和嚴重程度，但也要考慮受試者主訴的痛苦程度以及症狀對受試者生活品質影響的程度。進行這項評量時，要考慮到伴發症狀，如受試者主訴的吞嚥困難、舌的厚度等。

- 0 = 無。
- 1 = 可能肌肉有輕微僵硬、扭曲或異常姿勢。
- 2 = 輕度肌張力障礙。舌、頸部、四肢、軀幹輕度僵硬、扭曲或痙攣，或有輕度眼球上吊。受試者不一定會覺得痛苦。
- 3 = 中度肌張力障礙。肌肉中度僵硬、扭曲、收縮，或有中度眼球上吊。受試者常常說這些症狀使其感覺痛苦。希望迅速得到治療。
- 4 = 軀幹和/或四肢有重度肌張力障礙。由於有這些症狀，受試者的日常活動很困難，如吃飯和走路。迫切需要立即治療。

8 | 運動異常　Dyskinesia

　　異常運動過多。運動看起來明顯沒有目的，不規則，且不自主，見於臉部（臉部表情肌）、口部（口唇和口週邊區域）、舌、下頜、上肢（手臂、腕部、手、手指）、下肢（腿、膝部、踝部、腳趾）和/或軀幹（頸部、肩部、臀部）。要評量舞蹈症樣運動和手足徐動症樣運動，但不包括顫抖。評量的重點是客觀異常的不自主運動的發生頻率和嚴重程度，但也要考慮受試者主訴的痛苦程度以及症狀對受試者生活品質影響的程度。評量更多觀察到的自發運動障礙，而不是需要激發後出現的運動障礙。

- 0 = 無。
- 1 = 非特異性輕微的異常的不自主運動。局部間斷的，有輕度、異常的不自主運動。
- 2 = 局部持續有輕度、異常的不自主運動。≥2個部位間斷有輕度、異常的不自主運動，和/或局部間斷有中度、異常的不自主運動。
- 3 = 局部持續有中度、異常的不自主運動。≥2個部位間斷有中度、異常的不自主運動輕度，和/或局部間斷有重度、異常的不自主運動。
- 4 = 重度、異常的不自主運動。由於有這些症狀，受試者的日常活動比較困難。

9 | 整體嚴重程度　Overall severity

　　評量錐體外症狀的整體嚴重程度，既要考慮各項症狀的嚴重程度和發生頻率，也要考慮受試者主訴的痛苦程度，以及這些症狀對受試者日常活動影響的程度，還要考慮治療的必要性。

- 0 = 無。
- 1 = 輕微或不確定。
- 2 = 輕度。對受試者的日常活動幾乎沒有影響。不一定會感覺痛苦。
- 3 = 中度。對受試者的日常活動有一定程度的影響。常常會感覺痛苦。
- 4 = 重度。對受試者的日常活動有相當大的影響。感覺非常痛苦。

© Taiwanese version Shih-ku Lin, M.D./ English version Toshiya Inada, M.D.

Appendix III - Taiwanese version

DIEPSS（藥源性錐體外症狀評量表）所有項目評量表

研究：
病人：
評量者：
評量日期：　　　　年　　　月　　　日
評量時間：　　　　　　～

有關錨點分數的詳細說明，請熟讀DIEPSS評量員的評分手冊。

評分：
0 = 無，正常　None, Normal
1 = 輕微或不確定　Minimal, Questionable
2 = 輕度　Mild
3 = 中度　Moderate
4 = 重度　Severe

請圈出適當的一項

1　步態　Gait

步態拖曳、緩慢。評量步行速度減緩和步幅縮短的程度，手臂擺動減少的程度，前屈姿勢和前衝表現的程度。

Shuffling, slow gait. Evaluate the degree of reduction in speed and step, decrease in pendular arm movement, stooped posture and propulsion phenomenon.

0　1　2　3　4

2　運動遲緩　Bradykinesia

動作緩慢，活動很少：動作開始和/或結束比較遲緩，和/或有困難。評量臉部表情缺乏(面具臉)的程度，評量說話音腔單調、不清的程度。

Slowness and poverty of movements: Delay and/or difficulty in initiating and/or terminating movements. Rate degree of poverty of facial expression (mask-like face) and monotonous, slurred speech, as well.

0　1　2　3　4

3　流涎　Sialorrhea

唾液過多。

Excess salivation.

0　1　2　3　4

4　肌肉僵硬　Muscle rigidity

上臂屈伸運動有阻力。評量齒輪樣僵直、蠟樣屈曲、鉛管樣僵直以及腕關節的靈活度。

Resistance to flexion and extension of upper arms. Rate cogwheeling, waxy flexibility, lead-pipe rigidity and the degree of flexibility of wrists, as well.

0　1　2　3　4

5　顫抖　Tremor

反覆、有規則(4-8Hz)的節律性運動，見於口部、手指、四肢和軀幹這些部位。

Repetitive, regular (4-8 Hz), and rhythmic movements observed in the oral region, fingers, extremities, and trunk.

0　1　2　3　4

6　靜坐不能　Akathisia

主觀感覺坐立不安與相關痛苦；覺得坐不住，腿不停地動，忐忑不安，不停地想動等表現。還要評量運動增多的表現(身體搖晃、兩腳不停地換位、原地踏步、腿不停翹起來又放下、四處走動等)。

Subjective inner restlessness and related distress; awareness of the inability to remain seated, restless legs, fidgety feelings, desire to move constantly, etc. Rate increased motor phenomena (body rocking, shifting from foot to foot, stamping in place, crossing and uncrossing legs, pacing around, etc.), as well.

0　1　2　3　4

7　肌張力異常　Dystonia

肌張力亢奮誘發的症狀。肌肉僵硬、扭曲、持續方位異常，見于舌頭、頸部、四肢、軀幹等部位。評量吐舌、斜頸、頸後傾、牙關緊閉、眼球上吊、比薩症候群等表現。

Symptoms induced by the hypertonic state of muscles. Stiffness, twisting, and persistent abnormal position of muscles observed in tongue, neck, extremities, trunk, etc. Rate tongue protrusion, torticollis, retrocollis, trismus, oculogyric crisis, Pisa syndrome, etc.

0　1　2　3　4

8　運動異常　Dyskinesia

異常運動過多。運動看起來沒有目的，不規則，且不自主，見於臉部、口部、舌、下頜、四肢和/或軀幹。包括舞蹈症樣運動和手足徐動症樣運動，但不需評量顫抖。

Hyperkinetic abnormal movements. Apparently purposeless, irregular, and involuntary movements observed in face, mouth, tongue, jaw, extremities and/or trunk. Include choreic and athetoid movements, but do not rate tremor.

0　1　2　3　4

9　整體嚴重程度　Overall severity

錐體外症狀的整體嚴重程度。

Overall severity of extrapyramidal symptoms.

0　1　2　3　4

© Taiwanese version Shih-ku Lin, M.D./ English version Toshiya Inada, M.D.

Appendix IV - Korean version

DIEPSS(약물에 의한 추체외로 증상 평가 척도)평가자를 위한 지침서

이 척도는 항정신병 약물 치료를 하는 동안에 일어나는, 약물에 의한 추체외로 증상의 심각도를 평가하기 위해 만들어졌으며, 개별적 항목 8개와 포괄적 항목 1개로 구성되어 있다. 평가자는 의학 교육을 받은 사람으로서 신경학적 증상의 평가에 대한 충분한 지식이 있어야 한다. 또한 일관성 있는 자료를 얻기 위해 평가자는 이 척도의 사용 방법에 대한 충분한 훈련을 받아야 한다. 평가자는 주로 피검자와의 직접적인 인터뷰와, 인터뷰하는 동안의 관찰을 통하여 피검자의 증상을 평가해야 한다. 평가자는 또한 병실 근무자와 가족으로부터 얻은 정보도 참작해야 한다. 진전(tremor), 정좌불능증(akathisia), 근긴장이상(dystonia) 등의 개별 항목의 평가에서, 때때로 피검자는 인터뷰 기간보다는 밤에 약을 복용한 후 또는 잠들기 전과 같은 어느 일정한 때에만 그 증상들이 나타난다고 보고할 수도 있다. 이런 경우에, 평가자는 병실 근무자와 가족으로부터 얻은 정보뿐만 아니라 피검자와의 인터뷰도 고려하여 증상의 심각도를 신중하게 평가해야 한다. 개개의 연구 계획서에 정해진 평가 기간 동안에(예를 들면, 최근 24시간, 최근 3일 등) 관찰된 가장 심한 증상들을 평가해야 한다. 다음의 용어 해설은 특정한 항목의 평가를 위한 지침이다.

1 | 걸음걸이 Gait

피검자에게 평상시에 길을 걷는 것처럼 걸어 보라고 한다. 이 항목에서 걸음걸이의 느려짐을 평가한다. 즉, 팔을 앞뒤로 흔드는 진자 운동(pendular arm movement)의 감소와 더불어 걸음걸이 속도와 보폭의 감소 정도를 평가한다. 구부정한 자세와 전방돌진 현상(propulsion)의 정도도 고려한다. 이런 증상들의 강도가 기준점(anchor point)에 맞지 않으면, 피검자에게서 관찰되는 가장 심한 증상을 기준으로 평가한다. 걷기 시작하거나 멈출 때 나타나는 어려움의 정도는 운동완만(bradykinesia) 항목의 평가에도 고려해야 한다.

- 0 = 정상.
- 1 = 팔의 진자 운동이 최경도로 감소되며, 걸음걸이 속도와 보폭이 최경도로 감소됨.
- 2 = 팔의 진자 운동이 경도로 감소되며, 걸음걸이 속도와 보폭이 경도로 감소됨. 어떤 경우에는 경도의 구부정한 자세도 관찰됨.
- 3 = 팔의 진자 운동이 상당히 감소되며, 걸음걸이가 뚜렷이 늦어짐. 전형적인 구부정한 자세를 보이고 보폭이 좁아짐. 때때로 전방돌진 현상이 관찰됨.
- 4 = 혼자 걷기를 시작하는 것이 거의 불가능함. 걷기 시작한다 해도 팔의 진자 운동이 없고 보폭이 매우 좁으며, 발을 질질 끌면서 걷는 것이 관찰됨. 심한 전방돌진 현상이 관찰될 수 있음.

2 | 운동완만 Bradykinesia

운동의 느려짐과 빈약함으로 인해 활동이 감소된 것을 평가한다. 운동을 시작하는 것이 지연되고 때로는 어렵다. 얼굴 표정의 빈약한 정도(마스크 쓴 것 같은 얼굴)와 인터뷰 동안의 말투(단조롭고 명료하지 못한 말투)도 평가한다.

- 0 = 정상.
- 1 = 운동이 느려진 인상(impression).
- 2 = 경도의 운동완만. 운동이 느려지고 근긴장이 상실됨. 운동을 시작하거나 마칠 때 약간 지연됨. 말의 속도와 얼굴표정에서 경도의 감소를 보임.
- 3 = 중등도의 운동완만. 운동을 시작하거나 마칠 때 뚜렷한 장해가 있음. 중등도로 말의 속도가 느려지며, 중등도의 장해가 얼굴 표정에 나타남.
- 4 = 고도의 운동완만, 또는 무동증(akinesia). 거의 움직이지 않거나 움직일 때 많은 노력이 필요함. 얼굴 표정에 거의 변화가 없음(전형적인 마스크 쓴 것 같은 얼굴). 말이 현저하게 느려짐.

3 | 침흘림 Sialorrhea

과다한 타액 분비 정도를 평가한다.

- 0 = 정상.
- 1 = 최경도의 타액 분비 과다가 인터뷰하는 동안 관찰됨.
- 2 = 경도의 타액 고임이 인터뷰하는 동안 관찰됨. 말하는 데 어려움이 조금 있음.
- 3 = 중등도의 타액 분비 과다가 인터뷰하는 동안 관찰됨. 종종 말하기가 어려움.
- 4 = 고도의 타액 분비 과다가 항상 관찰되거나, 침을 입 밖으로 흘림(drooling).

4 | 근육 경직 Muscle rigidity

팔의 구부리기(flexion)와 펴기(extension)에 대한 저항의 심각도를 평가한다. 톱니바퀴현싱(cogwheeling), 손목의 굴곡성(flexibility) 정도, 납굴증(waxy flexibility)도 평가한다.

- 0 = 없음.
- 1 = 최경도의 저항을 보임.
- 2 = 경도의 저항을 보임. 때때로 경도의 톱니바퀴현상이 보임.
- 3 = 중등도의 저항을 보임. 명백한 톱니바퀴현상이 일어날 수 있 음.
- 4 = 극도의 저항을 보임. 동작이 중지되었을 때 한 자세를 그대로 유지하기도 함(납굴증). 극도의 근육 경직으로 인해 때때로 팔의 구부리기와 펴기가 불가능함.

5 | 진전 Tremor

입 부위, 손가락, 사지와 몸통에서 관찰되는 반복적이고, 규칙적 (4 –8 Hz)이며 주기적인 운동. 주로 객관적으로 관찰되는 증상의 빈도와 심각도에 중점을 두어 평가하지만, 피검자가 호소하는 고통의 정도, 그리고 증상으로 인하여 삶의 질에 영향을 받는 정도도 고려한다.

- 0 = 없음.
- 1 = 최경도의 비특이성 진전이 관찰되거나 또는 경도의 진전이 한 부위에서 간헐적으로 관찰됨.
- 2 = 경도의 진전이 한 부위에서 지속적으로 관찰됨. 경도의 진전이 두 부위 이상에서 간헐적으로 관찰되거나 또는 중등도의 진전이 한 부위에서 간헐적으로 관찰됨.
- 3 = 중등도의 진전이 한 부위에서 지속적으로 관찰됨. 중등도의 진전이 두 부위 이상에서 간헐적으로 관찰되거나 또는 고도의 진전이 한 부위에서 간헐적으로 관찰됨.
- 4 = 고도의 전신성(generalized) 진전 또는 전신 진전(whole body tremor).

6 | 정좌불능증 Akathisia

정좌불능증은 안절부절못하는 주관적인 느낌(subjective inner restlessness)과 객관적으로 증가된 운동 현상으로 이루어져 있다. 안절부절못하는 주관적인 느낌이란 앉아 있기가 불가능함, 안절부절못하는 다리(restless leg), 꼼지락거림(fidgetiness) 그리고 끊임없이 움직이려는 욕구 등을 자각(awareness)하는 것이다. 객관적으로 증가된 운동 현상이란 몸 흔들기(body rocking), 중심을 이 발 저 발로 옮기기(shifting from foot to foot), 제자리에서 발 구르기(stamping in place), 다리를 꼬았다 풀었다 하기(crossing and uncrossing legs), 주변을 왔다 갔다 하기(pacing around)와 같은 현상을 말한다. 주관적 증상의 심각도에 중점을 두어 평가하고, 증가된 운동 현상은 주관적 증상을 뒷받침하는 증거로 사용한다. 예를 들어, 안절부절못하는 느낌을 자각하지 않을 때는 0으로 평가한다. 정좌불능증의 특징적인 안절부절못하는 움직임이 관찰되더라도, 안절부절못하는 주관적인 느낌이 비특이적으로 명확하지 않게 있을 때는 1로 평가한다 (가성 정좌불능증(pseudoakathisia)). 정좌불능증의 평가에서는 검사 전반을 통해 나타나는 안절부절못함의 여부도 고려한다.

- 0 = 없음.
- 1 = 최경도의 비특이적인 안절부절못하는 느낌.
- 2 = 경도의 안절부절못하는 느낌을 자각하나 항상 고통스러운 것은 아님. 정좌불능증의 특징적인 증가된 운동 현상이 관찰될 수도 있음.
- 3 = 중등도의 안절부절못하는 느낌. 불편함과 고통스러움을 동반함. 안절부절못하는 주관적인 느낌으로 인해 유발되는 특징적인 다리의 안절부절못하는 움직임, 예를 들면 몸 흔들기, 중심을 이 발 저 발로 옮기기, 제자리에서 발 구르기와 같은 움직임이 관찰됨.
- 4 = 고도의 안절부절못하는 느낌. 자리에 앉아 있기가 불가능하거나 끊임없이 다리를 움직임. 수면 장애 또는 불안 상태를 일으킬 수 있는 명백히 고통스러운 상태임. 환자는 증상의 경감을 강력하게 원함.

7 | 근긴장이상 Dystonia

근긴장이상은 근육의 긴장과도 상태(hypertonic state)로 인해 유발되며, 혀, 목, 사지와 몸통 등에서 관찰되는 강직(stiffness), 꼬임(twisting), 연축(spasm), 수축(contraction), 그리고 지속적인 근육의 비정상적 위치(abnormal position)로 나타나는 증후군이다. 증상에는 혀 돌출(tongue protrusion), 사경(torticollis), 후굴성 사경(retrocollis), 턱관절경직(trismus), 안구운동발작(oculogyric crisis), 피사 증후군(Pisa syndrome) 등이 있다. 이 항목에서는 비정상적으로 증가된 근육 긴장의 정도만을 평가한다. 근긴장이상으로 인한 비정상 운동의 정도는 운동곤란증(dyskinesia)의 항목에서 평가해야 한다. 주로 객관적으로 관찰되는 증상의 빈도와 심각도에 중점을 두어 평가하지만, 피검자가 호소하는 고통의 정도와 증상으로 인하여 삶의 질에 영향을 받는 정도도 고려한다. 이 항목을 평가할 때 연하 곤란, 혀가 두꺼워짐(thickness of tongue) 등을 호소하는 것과 같은 동반된 증상도 고려한다.

0 = 없음.
1 = 최경도의 근육 당김(tightness), 꼬임, 또는 비정상적인 자세.
2 = 경도의 근긴장이상. 혀, 목, 사지, 몸통에서 경도의 강직, 꼬임, 연축이 관찰되거나 경도의 안구운동발작이 관찰됨. 항상 고통스러운 것은 아님.
3 = 중등도의 근긴장이상. 중등도의 강직, 꼬임, 수축 또는 안구운동발작이 관찰됨. 증상과 관련된 고통을 자주 호소함. 신속한 치료가 바람직함.
4 = 고도의 근긴장이상이 몸통 또는 사지에서 관찰됨. 이러한 증상 때문에 먹고 걷는 것과 같은 일상 활동이 현저히 어려움. 긴급한 치료가 필요함.

8 | 운동곤란증 Dyskinesia

비정상적인 과운동증. 명백하게 목적이 없고(purposeless) 불규칙적이며(irregular) 불수의적인(involuntary) 운동이 얼굴(얼굴 표정 근육), 입(입술과 입 주위), 혀, 턱, 상지(팔, 손목, 손, 손가락), 하지(다리, 무릎, 발목, 발가락), 또는 몸통(목, 어깨, 엉덩이)에서 관찰된다. 무도성(choreic) 및 무정위(athetoid) 운동을 평가하나 진전은 포함시키지 않는다. 주로 객관적으로 관찰된 비정상적인 불수의 운동의 빈도와 심각도에 중점을 두어 평가하지만, 피검자가 호소하는 고통의 정도와 증상으로 인하여 삶의 질에 영향을 받는 정도도 고려한다. 유발시켜 일어나는 운동은 자발적으로 관찰되는 운동보다 1점 낮게 평가한다.

0 = 없음.
1 = 최경도의 비특이적이고 비정상적인 불수의 운동이 관찰됨. 경도의 비정상적인 불수의 운동이 국한된 부위에서 간헐적으로 관찰됨.
2 = 경도의 비정상적인 불수의 운동이 국한된 부위에서 지속적으로 관찰됨. 경도의 비정상적인 불수의 운동이 두 부위 이상에서 간헐적으로 관찰되거나 또는 중등도의 비정상적인 불수의 운동이 국한된 부위에서 간헐적으로 관찰됨.
3 = 중등도의 비정상적인 불수의 운동이 국한된 부위에서 지속적으로 관찰됨. 중등도의 비정상적인 불수의 운동이 두 부위 이상에서 간헐적으로 관찰되거나 또는 고도의 비정상적인 불수의 운동이 국한된 부위에서 간헐적으로 관찰됨.
4 = 고도의 비정상적인 불수의 운동이 관찰됨. 증상으로 인해 일상 활동에 어려움이 있음.

9 | 전체적 심각도 Overall severity

추체외로 증상의 전체적 심각도는 개별 증상들의 심각도와 빈도, 피검자가 호소하는 고통의 정도, 증상으로 인해 일상 활동에 영향을 받는 정도와 치료가 필요한 정도를 고려하여 평가한다.

0 = 없음.
1 = 최경도 또는 의심스러운 정도.
2 = 경도. 피검자의 일상 활동에 거의 영향을 주지 않음. 항상 고통스럽지는 않음.
3 = 중등도. 피검자의 일상 활동에 어느 정도 영향을 미침. 자주 고통스러움.
4 = 고도. 피검자의 일상 활동에 심각한 영향을 미침. 매우 고통스러움.

© Korean version Yong Sik Kim, M.D./ English version Toshiya Inada, M.D.

Appendix IV - Korean version

DIEPSS(약물에 의한 추체외로 증상 평가 척도)전 항목평가 용지

연구 (Study) :	코드 (Code)
환자명 (Patient) :	0 =없음,정상 None, Normal
평가자 (Rater) :	1 =극히 경증, 불확실 Minimal, Questionable
평가일시 (Date of evaluation) : 년 월 일	2 =경증 Mild
평가 시간 (Time of evaluation) : ~	3 =중등도 Moderate
	4 =중증 Severe

엥커 포인트의 상세한 설명에 대해서는, DIEPSS의 평가자용 매뉴얼을 숙독할 것.
Read the rater's manual of DIEPSS carefully, for detailed explanation of anchor points.

적당한 평점에 ○을 붙여 주세요.(Circle one as appropriate.)

1 걸음걸이 Gait
속도와 보폭, 팔흔들기, 구부정한 자세, 보폭, 전방돌진 현상.
Shuffling, slow gait. Evaluate the degree of reduction in speed and step, decrease in pendular arm movement, stooped posture and propulsion phenomenon.

0 1 2 3 4

2 운동완만 Bradykinesia
느려진 움직임, 운동 시작/종료의 어려움, 표정 감소, 말의 속도 및 말투.
Slowness and poverty of movements: Delay and/or difficulty in initiating and/or terminating movements. Rate degree of poverty of facial expression (mask-like face) and monotonous, slurred speech, as well.

0 1 2 3 4

3 침흘림 Sialorrhea
과다한 타액 분비 정도를 평가한다.
Excess salivation.

0 1 2 3 4

4 근육 경직 Muscle rigidity
상지의 구부리기/펴기 시의 저항감 및 톱니바퀴현상, 납굴증도 평가한다.
Resistance to flexion and extension of upper arms. Rate cogwheeling, waxy flexibility, lead-pipe rigidity and the degree of flexibility of wrists, as well.

0 1 2 3 4

5 진전 Tremor
입 부위, 손가락, 사지와 몸통에서 관찰되는 반복적이고, 규칙적 (4 –8 Hz)이며 주기적인 운동.
Repetitive, regular (4-8 Hz), and rhythmic movements observed in the oral region, fingers, extremities, and trunk.

0 1 2 3 4

6 정좌불능증 Akathisia
아래의 주관적 소견/특징적 운동[앉아서 – 서서]을 평가.
*주관적 느낌: 앉아있지 못하겠다, 안절부절못하는 다리, 꼼지락거림, 계속 움직이고싶은 욕구.
*특징적 운동: (앉아서) 상체 흔들기, 다리 꼬기–풀기.
 (서서) 발을 쿵쿵, 몸무게를 이쪽–저쪽 다리로 자주 옮김, 종종걸음.
Subjective inner restlessness and related distress; awareness of the inability to remain seated, restless legs, fidgety feelings, desire to move constantly, etc. Rate increased motor phenomena (body rocking, shifting from foot to foot, stamping in place, crossing and uncrossing legs, pacing around, etc.), as well.

0 1 2 3 4

7 근긴장이상 Dystonia
근긴장이상은 근육의 긴장과도 상태로 인해 유발되며, 혀, 목, 사지와 몸통 등에서 관찰되는 강직, 꼬임, 연축, 수축, 그리고 지속적인 근육의 비정상적 위치로 나타나는 증후군이다. 증상에는 혀 돌출, 사경, 후굴성 사경, 턱관절경직, 안구운동발작, 피사 증후군 등이 있다.
Symptoms induced by the hypertonic state of muscles. Stiffness, twisting, and persistent abnormal position of muscles observed in tongue, neck, extremities, trunk, etc. Rate tongue protrusion, torticollis, retrocollis, trismus, oculogyric crisis, Pisa syndrome, etc.

0 1 2 3 4

8 운동곤란증 Dyskinesia
비정상적인 과운동증. 명백하게 목적이 없고 불규칙적이며 불수의적인 운동이 얼굴(얼굴 표정 근육), 입(입술과 입 주위), 혀, 턱, 상지(팔, 손목, 손, 손가락), 하지(다리, 무릎, 발목,발가락), 또는 몸통(목, 어깨, 엉덩이)에서 관찰된다. 무도성 및 무정위 운동을 평가하나 진전은 포함시키지 않는다.
Hyperkinetic abnormal movements. Apparently purposeless, irregular, and involuntary movements observed in face, mouth, tongue, jaw, extremities and/or trunk. Include choreic and athetoid movements, but do not rate tremor.

0 1 2 3 4

9 전체적 심각도 Overall severity
추체외로 증상의 전체적 심각도.
Overall severity of extrapyramidal symptoms.

0 1 2 3 4

© Korean version Yong Sik Kim, M.D./ English version Toshiya Inada, M.D.

Appendix V - English version

DIEPSS (Drug-induced Extrapyramidal Symptoms Scale) Rater's Manual

This scale is designed to evaluate the severity of drug-induced extrapyramidal symptoms occurring during antipsychotic drug treatment, and consists of 8 individual items and 1 global item. Raters should have medical training and have sufficient knowledge of the evaluation of neurological symptoms. They also need to have sufficient training on how to use this scale so that they can reproduce stable data. Raters should evaluate the subject's symptoms principally from direct interview with the subject and from observations during the interview. Raters should also take information obtained from the ward personnel and from relatives into consideration. In evaluating individual items of tremor, akathisia, dystonia, etc., the subject may sometimes report that the symptoms appear only at certain times other than during the evaluation interview, such as after receiving night medication or before sleep. In such cases, the raters should carefully evaluate the severity of symptoms considering the interview with the subject as well as the information obtained from the ward personnel and relatives. The severest symptoms observed within the rating period determined in the individual research protocols (e.g. recent 24 hours, recent 3 days, etc.) should be considered for evaluation. The following glossary represents guidelines for rating the specific items.

1 | Gait

Ask the subject to walk as he/she normally would on the street. Rate slowness of gait in this item, namely, the degree of reduction in speed and step, as well as decrease in pendular arm movement. Also consider the degree of stooped posture and propulsion phenomenon. When the intensity of these symptoms does not fit an anchor point, rate giving priority to the severest symptom observed in the subject. The degree of difficulty in initiating and/or terminating walking should also be considered in rating the item of bradykinesia.

0 = Normal.

1 = Impression of minimal reduction in speed and step of gait, and minimal decrease in pendular arm movements.

2 = Mild reduction in speed and step of gait with mild decrease in pendular arm movements. Mild stooped posture is also observed in some cases.

3 = Clearly slowed gait with greatly diminished pendular arm movements. Typical stooped posture and gait with small steps. Propulsion phenomenon is sometimes observed.

4 = Initiation of walking alone is barely possible. Even if gait is initiated, the subject shows shuffling gait with very small steps and no pendular arm movements are observed. Severe propulsion phenomenon may be observed.

2 | Bradykinesia

Reduced activity due to slowness and poverty of movements. Initiating movements is delayed and is sometimes difficult. Rate the degree of poverty of facial expression (mask-like face) and speech during interview (monotonous, slurred speech), as well.

0 = Normal.

1 = Impression of slowness in movements.

2 = Mild bradykinesia. Slowed movements and loss of muscle tone. Slight delay in initiation and/or termination of movements. Mild reduction in facial expression and rate of speech.

3 = Moderate bradykinesia. Clear impairment in initiating and/or terminating movements. Rate of speech is moderately slowed, and facial expression is moderately impaired.

4 = Severe bradykinesia, or akinesia. The subject rarely moves, or moves with great effort. Almost no changes in facial expression (typical mask like face). Markedly slowed speech.

3 | Sialorrhea

Rate the severity of excess salivation.

0 = Normal.

1 = Impression of minimal excess salivation during interview.

2 = Mild excess saliva pooling in mouth observed during interview. Little difficulty in speaking.

3 = Moderate excess salivation observed during interview. Often results in difficulty in speaking.

4 = Constantly observed severe excess salivation or drooling.

4 | Muscle rigidity

Rate the severity of resistance to flexion and extension of the arms. Rate cogwheeling, waxy flexibility, and the degree of flexibility of wrists, as well.

0 = Absent.

1 = Impression of minimal resistance to flexion and extension of the arms.

2 = Mild resistance to flexion and extension of the arms. Mild cogwheeling is sometimes noted.

3 = Moderate resistance to flexion and extension of the arms. Obvious cogwheeling may occur.

4 = Extreme resistance to flexion and extension of the arms. The subject may maintain posture, when interrupted (waxy flexibility). Flexion and extension of the arms is sometimes impossible due to extreme muscle rigidity.

5 | Tremor

Repetitive, regular (4-8 Hz), and rhythmic movements observed in the oral region, fingers, extremities, and trunk. Rate principally giving greater weight to the frequency and the severity of the symptoms observed objectively, however, consider the degree of distress that the subject complains of and that of the effects on the subject's quality of life due to the symptoms, as well.

0 = Absent.

1 = Non-specific minimal tremor, and/or mild tremor observed intermittently in a single area.

2 = Mild tremor is observed persistently in a single area. Mild tremor in two or more regions and/or moderate tremor in a single area are observed intermittently.

3 = Moderate tremor is observed persistently in a single area. Moderate tremor in two or more regions and/or severe tremor in a single area are observed intermittently.

4 = Severe generalized tremor, and/or whole body tremor.

6 | Akathisia

Akathisia consists of subjective inner restlessness, such as awareness of the inability to remain seated, restless legs, fidgetiness, and the desire to move constantly, and of objective increased motor phenomena, such as body rocking, shifting from foot to foot, stamping in place, crossing and uncrossing legs, pacing around. Rate giving greater weight to the severity of subjective symptoms and use the increased motor phenomena as evidence to support subjective symptoms. For example, rate 0 when no awareness of inner restlessness is observed, and rate 1 when only non-specific indefinite inner restlessness is obtained, even if characteristic restless movements of akathisia are observed (pseudoakathisia). In rating akathisia, consider the presence or absence of restlessness throughout the entire examination, as well.

0 = Absent.

1 = Non-specific minimal inner restlessness.

2 = Awareness of mild inner restlessness not always resulting in subjective distress. Characteristic increased motor phenomena of akathisia may be observed.

3 = Moderate inner restlessness. Results in uncomfortable symptoms and distress. Characteristic restless movements of the legs derived from the subjective inner restlessness, such as body rocking, shifting from foot to foot and stamping in place, are observed.

4 = Severe inner restlessness. Results in the inability to remain seated, or moving the legs constantly. Obviously distressing condition which may induce disturbed sleep and/or anxiety states. Subject strongly desires relief of symptoms.

7 | Dystonia

Dystonia is a syndrome induced by the hypertonic state of muscles, manifested by stiffness, twisting, spasms, contraction, and persistent abnormal position of muscles observed in the tongue, neck, extremities, trunk, etc. Symptoms include tongue protrusion, torticollis, retrocollis, trismus, oculogyric crisis, Pisa syndrome, etc. Rate only the abnormal degree of increased muscle tone on this item. The degree of abnormal movements resulting from dystonia should be rated in the item of dyskinesia. Rate principally giving greater weight to the frequency and the severity of symptoms observed objectively, however, consider the degree of distress that the subject complains of and that of the effects on the subject's quality of life due to the symptoms, as well. Take the concomitant symptoms into consideration in rating this item, such as the subject's complaint of difficulty in swallowing, thickness of the tongue, etc.

0 = Absent.

1 = Impression of minimal muscle tightness, twisting or abnormal posture.

2 = Mild dystonia. Mild stiffness, twisting or spasms observed in tongue, neck, extremities, trunk, or mild oculogyric crisis. The subject does not always feel distress.

3 = Moderate dystonia. Moderate stiffness, twisting, contraction or oculogyric crisis. The subject often complains of distress related to the symptoms. Prompt treatment is desirable.

4 = Severe dystonia observed in trunk and/or extremities. The subject has marked difficulties with activities of daily living, such as eating and walking, due to these symptoms. Urgent treatment is indicated.

8 | Dyskinesia

Hyperkinetic abnormal movements. Apparently purposeless, irregular, and involuntary movements observed in face (muscles of facial expression), mouth (lips and perioral area), tongue, jaw, upper extremity (arms, wrists, hands, fingers), lower extremity (legs, knees, ankles, toes) and/or trunk (neck, shoulders, hips). Choreic and athetoid movements are rated, but tremor is not included. Rate principally giving greater weight to the frequency and the severity of abnormal involuntary movements observed objectively, however, consider the degree of distress that the subject complains of and that of the effects on the subject's quality of life due to the symptoms, as well. Rate movements that occur upon activation one less than those observed spontaneously.

0 = Absent.

1 = Non-specific minimal abnormal involuntary movements are observed. Mild abnormal involuntary movements are observed intermittently in a localized area.

2 = Mild abnormal involuntary movements are observed persistently in a localized area. Mild abnormal involuntary movements in two or more regions and/or moderate abnormal involuntary movements in a localized area are observed intermittently.

3 = Moderate abnormal involuntary movements are observed persistently in a localized area. Moderate abnormal involuntary movements in two or more regions and/or severe abnormal involuntary movements in a localized area are observed intermittently.

4 = Severe abnormal involuntary movements are observed. The subject has difficulty with activities of daily living due to the symptoms.

9 | Overall severity

Rate overall severity of extrapyramidal symptoms, considering the severity and the frequency of individual symptoms, the degree of distress that the subject complains of, that of the effects on the subject's activities of daily living due to the symptoms, and that of the necessity for their treatments.

0 = Absent.

1 = Minimal or questionable.

2 = Mild. Hardly affects the subject's activities of daily living. Not always feels distress.

3 = Moderate. Affects the subject's activities of daily living to some degree. Often feels distress.

4 = Severe. Affects the subject's activities of daily living significantly. Strongly feels distress.

© Toshiya INADA, M.D.

Appendix V - English version

DIEPSS (Drug-induced Extrapyramidal Symptoms Scale) Evaluation Sheet for All Items

Study:	Code:
Patient:	0 = None, Normal
Rater:	1 = Minimal, Questionable
Date of evaluation: Mo. Day Yr.	2 = Mild
Time of evaluation: ∼	3 = Moderate
Read the rater's manual of DIEPSS carefully, for detailed explanation of anchor points.	4 = Severe

Circle one as appropriate.

1 Gait
Shuffling, slow gait. Evaluate the degree of reduction in speed and step, decrease in pendular arm movement, stooped posture and propulsion phenomenon.   0 1 2 3 4

2 Bradykinesia
Slowness and poverty of movements: Delay and/or difficulty in initiating and/or terminating movements. Rate degree of poverty of facial expression (mask-like face) and monotonous, slurred speech, as well.   0 1 2 3 4

3 Sialorrhea
Excess salivation.   0 1 2 3 4

4 Muscle rigidity
Resistance to flexion and extension of upper arms. Rate cogwheeling, waxy flexibility, lead-pipe rigidity and the degree of flexibility of wrists, as well.   0 1 2 3 4

5 Tremor
Repetitive, regular (4-8 Hz), and rhythmic movements observed in the oral region, fingers, extremities, and trunk.   0 1 2 3 4

6 Akathisia
Subjective inner restlessness and related distress; awareness of the inability to remain seated, restless legs, fidgety feelings, desire to move constantly, etc. Rate increased motor phenomena (body rocking, shifting from foot to foot, stamping in place, crossing and uncrossing legs, pacing around, etc.), as well.   0 1 2 3 4

7 Dystonia
Symptoms induced by the hypertonic state of muscles. Stiffness, twisting, and persistent abnormal position of muscles observed in tongue, neck, extremities, trunk, etc. Rate tongue protrusion, torticollis, retrocollis, trismus, oculogyric crisis, Pisa syndrome, etc.   0 1 2 3 4

8 Dyskinesia
Hyperkinetic abnormal movements. Apparently purposeless, irregular, and involuntary movements observed in face, mouth, tongue, jaw, extremities and/or trunk. Include choreic and athetoid movements, but do not rate tremor.   0 1 2 3 4

9 Overall severity
Overall severity of extrapyramidal symptoms.   0 1 2 3 4

© Toshiya INADA, M.D.